HOW TO REACH & TEACH STUDENTS with DYSLEXIA

CYNTHIA M. STOWE

THE CENTER FOR APPLIED RESEARCH IN EDUCATION
West Nyack, New York 10994

Library of Congress Cataloging-in-Publication Data

Stowe, Cynthia.
How to reach & teach students with dyslexia / Cynthia M. Stowe.
p. cm.
Includes bibliographical references.
USBN 0-13-013571-2
1. Dyslexics—Education. 2. Dyslexia. I. Title. II. Title: How to reach and teach students with dyslexia.

LCA4708.S86 2000
371.91′44 21—dc21 99-045662

Acquisitions Editor: *Susan Kolwicz*
Production Editor: *Tom Curtin*
Interior Design/Formatter: *Dee Coroneos*

Printed in the United States of America

10 9 8 7 6 5 4 3 2 1

ISBN 0-13-013571-2

THE CENTER FOR APPLIED RESEARCH IN EDUCATION
West Nyack, NY 10994

On the World Wide Web at http://www.PHedu.com

DEDICATION

This book is dedicated to the people who spoke about their experiences with dyslexia with such eloquence and courage:

Daniel
Fran
Helen
Jeremiah
Mike
Mya
Naomi
Rafael
Sonia
Thomas

Although these aren't their real names, they know who they are.

ACKNOWLEDGMENTS

I wish to thank the following people.

- Robert Stowe, for his love and support
- Hedy Christenson, for all the practical help which she gave me on this book and, also, for being such a wonderful colleague and friend
- Cynthia Conway Waring, dear friend, for encouraging me to write this book and for supporting me throughout it
- Susan Kolwicz, my editor, for believing in me, and for her constant support and help
- Jean-Marie Aubin, for her enthusiasm and support
- Dr. Peter B. Martin, for sharing his expertise
- Chris Brunaccioni, for sharing information and books
- Michael Daley, Jessie Haas, Jean Shaw, and Nancy Hope Wilson: encouragers and critiquers all
- The International Dyslexia Association: a dedicated voice of advocacy

ABOUT THE AUTHOR

Cynthia Stowe has worked with students with dyslexia for over thirty years, as a classroom teacher, a school psychologist, and a special education teacher. She has worked mostly in public schools but has also taught in private schools for students with dyslexia, in literacy programs for adults, and in clinic settings. She currently works as a consulting school psychologist at a school for children with special needs and as a consulting teacher at a local literacy program for adults. She also has a private tutoring practice for students with dyslexia.

Cynthia is the author of

- *Spelling Smart! A Ready-to-Use Activities Program for Students with Spelling Difficulties* (The Center for Applied Research in Education, 1996) and
- *Let's Write! A Ready-to-Use Activities Program for Students with Special Needs* (The Center for Applied Research in Education, 1997).

In addition, she has written three novels for children:

- *Home Sweet Home, Good-bye* (Scholastic Hardcover, 1990).
- *Dear Mom, in Ohio for a Year* (Scholastic Hardcover, 1992).
- *Not-so-normal, Norman* (Albert Whitman and Company, 1995).

ABOUT THIS RESOURCE

THE PLACE: a fourth-grade classroom in a small rural school

THE TIME: more than 30 years ago

THE MAIN CHARACTER: a boy who stands at least a foot taller than his peers. He has been retained twice already, so his height is as much due to his older age as it is to genetics. He cannot read or write or spell very well. He manages with mathematics. He is obviously intelligent, because he can talk about many different things. He is particularly interested in basketball, and he avidly follows a local university team.

ANOTHER MAIN CHARACTER: the boy's teacher. She knows that the boy is smart, but no one at the small school can tell her anything about why he is not learning. Her training has taught her only to work with "typical" children. She tries to help him, but he learns very little in his fourth-grade year. She talks with him a lot about basketball. She is grateful that he doesn't seem too unhappy at school.

This boy really existed, and the author of this resource was his teacher. She was so concerned about her own lack of understanding about why he wasn't learning that she began to seek out information. That quest led her to become a school psychologist and special education teacher. In time, she decided that the boy most probably had dyslexia.

Dyslexia is a learning style with strengths and weaknesses that require appropriate intervention. When effective instruction is provided, students with dyslexia can flourish and learn. Because of their great strengths, they can be very successful in their own careers. They can also contribute a great deal to our society.

A teacher *does* have to understand what dyslexia is, however, and how to provide appropriate instruction. *How to Reach and Teach Students with Dyslexia* gives you the information you need. It details the characteristics of this learning style and how accurate diagnosis can be made. It describes techniques that can be used to teach the student with dyslexia. Chapters on associated issues such as ADD and ADHD, emotional and social concerns, and important times of transition are also included.

Basic beliefs about dyslexia presented in this resource are the following:

- The student with dyslexia generally has average to above average intellectual potential.

- It is a myth that more males than females have dyslexia. Current research is showing that as many females as males have this learning style.
- Dyslexia is a learning style that people are born with. They do nothing to cause it.
- People do not grow out of dyslexia. Appropriate instruction is needed for success with reading, writing, spelling, math, and the other academic subjects.
- If a person has dyslexia, there is nothing wrong with her brain. She simply learns subjects such as reading and spelling by a different method.
- Dyslexia is not contagious. It is now generally believed to be a genetically based condition which tends to occur in families.
- Dyslexia is not just about reversing letters and numbers. It is primarily a language issue, affecting phonemic awareness and language processing. It can also affect other skills such as fine motor functioning.
- If a person has dyslexia, he can have different degrees of the learning style.
- Dyslexia affects each person differently. Most people with dyslexia have difficulty with decoding words when reading, but some do not.
- There are some common weaknesses. For example, spelling is almost always a challenging task. With proper instruction, people with dyslexia *can* become competent spellers, especially when they learn to use a spell checker on a computer.
- Learning a foreign language can be hard. Some colleges waive language requirements for students with dyslexia.
- Testing situations—especially timed testing—are generally difficult.
- Significant strengths are often associated with dyslexia. These commonly include excellent creative thinking, the ability to see patterns in a mass of data, the ability to concentrate and focus intently on a challenging and interesting task, and artistic and musical talents.
- Many famous people, like Thomas Edison and Albert Einstein, are believed to have had dyslexia.
- The student with dyslexia *can* go to college. She may need some support and special accommodations, but she can be successful with higher education. In fact, some students with dyslexia, once they reach college, succeed brilliantly, because they can finally choose to work and study in their areas of strength and interest.
- Most important: *Students with dyslexia are not stupid. They experience failure because the wrong teaching methods were used. Once the proper teaching methods are used, they can be successful with academics.*

It is a challenge to work with students with dyslexia; it is also a great privilege. They are amazing people who can, and do, offer much to the world. The following is a brief description of the chapters in this book:

- Chapter 1, *What Is Dyslexia?*, provides a definition of dyslexia. It describes characteristics of this learning style and lists some of the important issues that can be associated with it. A major focus of the chapter is to talk about strengths which people with dyslexia often have. This is included because strengths are as important to consider as weaknesses when teaching students with dyslexia.
- Chapter 2, *Assessment and Diagnosis*, deals with the critically important topic of testing. This area can be confusing, because students with dyslexia can have different degrees of the learning style (from very mild to significant). They can also have different constellations of characteristics. There are, however, some important diagnostic signs of dyslexia, and a skilled diagnostician can be extremely helpful in the initial stages of planning an appropriate program.
- Chapter 3, *About Special Education*, gives basic information about special education, including the referral process, team meetings and IEPs. The relevant federal laws are cited. The chapter ends with suggestions for teachers and parents on how to help get appropriate services for students.
- Chapter 4, *Intervention*, discusses how to decide how much specialized instruction is needed for a student, and where that instruction can be provided: in the regular classroom, with an individual tutor, in a resource room, in a self-contained class for students with nontraditional learning styles, or in a special school. In addition, some specialists who can offer help are described.
- Chapter 5, *Ten General Principles of Instruction*, outlines ten important basics for teaching students with dyslexia. These include using multisensory teaching methods, presenting material sequentially, and presenting material in small units. These general principles apply to all areas of instruction.
- Chapter 6, *Teaching Reading*, discusses in depth how to teach reading to students with dyslexia. It covers all levels, from the student who doesn't know letter names and sounds to the student who decodes well but who needs help with reading comprehension. The issue of whether to use phonics or whole-language instruction is raised, and the conclusion is to integrate both. Teaching the structure of the English language is critically important for students with dyslexia, but they also need to practice thinking about what they are reading.
- Chapter 7, *Teaching Handwriting*, describes basic principles of instruction. Whereas there are very few students who have dysgraphia, many students with dyslexia need specialized instruction in this area. They profit from having their large arm muscles inform their small finger muscles. It also helps them to associate simple language cues with letter formation, and to learn the letters in groups of similar beginning strokes.

- Chapter 8, *Teaching Spelling,* discusses how to teach this very important academic skill. Most students with dyslexia have difficulty with spelling. A teaching approach which integrates phonics instruction with whole language philosophy is recommended. Thus, students utilize patterns in the English language, rather than having to memorize hundreds of isolated words. As they are doing this, they learn about the history of the language, and they, also, enjoy working with their spelling patterns.

- Chapter 9, *Teaching Writing,* offers a structured approach to this necessary skill that is so often difficult for students with dyslexia. The basics of word, sentence, and paragraph writing are discussed, and then the more advanced skills of essay and report writing. The focus is on developing independence and enjoyment of writing.

- Chapter 10, *Teaching Math,* provides a method that utilizes a multisensory, hands-on approach. Emphasis is placed on arithmetic, since so many students with dyslexia have difficulties with the numerical calculations of addition, subtraction, multiplication and division. Once students have mastered these basics, however, they often go on to achieve great success with more advanced mathematical concepts.

- Chapter 11, *Teaching Related Subjects,* talks about how the ten general principles of instruction that are presented in Chapter 5 are relevant to the teaching of Social Studies, Science, Art, Music and Physical Education. The challenging areas of homework and testing are also discussed.

- In Chapter 12, *Teaching Everyday Skills,* the issues of time, money, the memory for important details such as phone numbers, dealing with environmental print such as job applications, and keeping track of possessions are examined. Competency in these skills are particularly important, because they are needed in real life situations. Without competency, students with dyslexia are at a disadvantage with these necessary life skills, and can be easily embarrassed.

- In Chapter 13, *Issues Related to Dyslexia,* three areas in which people with dyslexia can have difficulties are discussed. These are: speech and language skills, gross motor skills, and fine motor skills. The types of possible problems are presented, as well as descriptions of professionals who can offer help. Suggestions are given for ways in which teachers can be supportive.

- Chapter 14, *ADD and ADHD,* discusses these challenging conditions, since many students with dyslexia also experience symptoms of them. Characteristics are described, and suggestions for ways that teachers can help are offered. There is a brief discussion of medication and alternatives to medication.

- Chapter 15, *Behavior and Social Skills,* presents fictional profiles of three types of students with behavioral issues: a student with impulsive and acting out behaviors; a student with withdrawn, isolating, and passive resistive behaviors;

and a student with off-target behaviors. Suggestions for ways that teachers can help are offered.

- Chapter 16, *Self Esteem and Other Emotional Needs*, discusses the critically important area of how people with dyslexia feel about themselves. Because most begin their academic careers with traditional curriculum, they experience a great deal of failure. They, thus, often define themselves as less intelligent than their peers. Also, people with dyslexia usually have surprising strengths as well as surprising weaknesses. This makes it difficult for other people to understand them. Some ways that teachers can help are offered.
- In Chapter 17, *Transitions*, the transition from elementary to middle school and junior high, the transition into high school, and the transitions into trade or technical school, college, and the world of work are discussed. The important issue of remediation versus accommodation is examined. Ways that teachers can help are offered.
- Chapter 18, *What Can Parents Do?,* helps teachers assist parents and guardians in their critically important roles. Four main areas are covered: learning how to observe, providing names of informational resources, giving suggestions for encouraging academic growth at home, and giving suggestions in problem areas such as homework and social and emotional issues. Parents and teachers are a team. This chapter helps them work effectively as one.
- Chapter 19, *Talents,* deals with the very important area of strengths. Information is given on how to help students discover their talents and, then, how to assist students to utilize them in the classroom. Both students and our society need these good abilities.
- Chapter 20, *The Adult with Dyslexia*, begins with an interview, because all adults with dyslexia have a story to tell about their educational histories. All too often, this is a story of frustration. This chapter provides insight into interacting with adults with dyslexia. It also offers specific suggestions for ways to teach them, if they wish to pursue instruction. The chapter ends with a discussion of college.

There are excerpts from interviews in every chapter of this book. Pseudonyms are used throughout, even with professionals and other people who are mentioned. All of the people interviewed have had a great deal of personal experience with dyslexia. Most of them have this fascinating learning style. They tell their stories eloquently and with great courage. Listen to their stories and learn from their wisdom.

CONTENTS

CHAPTER 3
ABOUT SPECIAL EDUCATION

CHAPTER 4
INTERVENTION

CHAPTER 5
TEN GENERAL PRINCIPLES OF INSTRUCTION

Chapter 6
TEACHING READING

CHAPTER 7

TEACHING HANDWRITING

CHAPTER 8

TEACHING SPELLING

CHAPTER 9

TEACHING WRITING

Chapter 10
TEACHING MATH

CHAPTER 11
TEACHING RELATED SUBJECTS

CHAPTER 12
TEACHING EVERYDAY SKILLS

CHAPTER 13

ISSUES RELATED TO DYSLEXIA

CHAPTER 14
ADD AND ADHD

CHAPTER 15
BEHAVIOR AND SOCIAL SKILLS

CHAPTER 16

SELF-ESTEEM AND OTHER EMOTIONAL NEEDS

CHAPTER 17

TRANSITIONS

CHAPTER 18
WHAT CAN PARENTS DO?

CHAPTER 19
TALENTS

CHAPTER 20

THE ADULT WITH DYSLEXIA

CHAPTER 1

WHAT IS DYSLEXIA?

Dyslexia is a learning style with strengths and with weaknesses that require appropriate intervention. When this instruction is provided, students can learn. The following are important principles:

- People with dyslexia can learn and can become very successful in school and in life.
- It is never too late for proper instruction.
- Many strengths and gifts often exist as a part of this learning style. These are as important to consider as the weaknesses.

Dyslexia affects a person's ability to deal with language, including spoken language as well as written. A person with dyslexia can have difficulty understanding, remembering, organizing and using verbal symbols. Because of this, many basic skills can be affected, especially reading and writing, spelling, handwriting, and arithmetic. In addition, other issues can occur concurrently with dyslexia.

DEFINITIONS

There are hundreds and possibly thousands of definitions of dyslexia.

A serious and complete definition was adopted by the Orton Dyslexia society, renamed The International Dyslexia Association, an organization devoted to helping people with dyslexia, in 1994. This organization states:

> Dyslexia is a neurologically based, often familial disorder which interferes with the acquisition and processing of language. Varying in degrees of severity, it is manifested by difficulties in receptive and expressive language—including phonological processing—in reading, writing, spelling, handwriting, and sometimes in arithmetic. Dyslexia is not a result of lack of motivation, sensory impairment, inadequate instructional or environmental opportunities, or other limiting conditions, but may

> occur together with these conditions. Although dyslexia is lifelong, individuals with dyslexia frequently respond successfully to timely and appropriate intervention.*

This definition is compact and contains a great deal of information and beliefs about dyslexia that are shared by this writer. To restate, dyslexia is not based on emotional or environmental factors but is a neurologically based condition that often occurs in families. Its level of severity varies widely among individuals. It affects language in general, and therefore the academic areas where language is involved, especially reading and written language. Occasionally mathematics is also affected. Even though poor teaching does not cause dyslexia, appropriate instruction can greatly help. Dyslexia can occur concurrently with other conditions, such as ADD or ADHD, and people do not outgrow it.

Definitions help us understand this perplexing and interesting condition, but we get a more vibrant picture, and perhaps the best "definition," when we think of individuals. Imagine a little boy who is a first-grader. Let's call him Harry. He seemed bright and normal as a toddler, a little active perhaps, but he responded well to structure and limits. His parents, Sonia and Michael, learned to be careful with his diet and not to feed him much junk food, because he seemed to get hyperactive when he ate a lot of sugar. Harry learned to walk on time and to speak, and he got along well with other kids. He did seem a little young for his age, so Sonia and Michael kept him home an extra year, especially because he had a summer birthday.

When Harry got to kindergarten, his teachers liked him a great deal, and he had fun at school. He couldn't seem to learn his letters or his numbers, however, and he was a little reluctant to enter first grade. All that year, Sonia and Michael worked with Harry, using flashcards with letters for drill. Night after night, he copied spelling words in a light and wobbly hand, reversing letters and just not getting the shapes correct.

At school, Harry's teachers knew that he was trying. They gave him extra time to finish projects and even worked with him at recess to help him catch up. They tried not to do that too often, however, because Harry was good at games and the other kids liked him. He needed his recesses, but he also needed so much extra help. It was hard to know what to do. At the end of first grade, his teacher referred him for an evaluation of his needs. "I know that Harry is a very bright boy," she wrote on the referral form, "but he just isn't achieving up to his potential."

There are so many stories of students like Harry, and we will tell some of them in this book. We will also attempt to provide the best current information on how to teach them.

---

*A definition of dyslexia, adopted by the Orton Dyslexic Society, now known as the International Dyslexic Association. Used by permission. The International Dyslexia Association has also published an additional, more technical definition of dyslexia for use within the research community.

CHARACTERISTICS ASSOCIATED WITH DYSLEXIA

People are often very confused by dyslexia, because it occurs in such different forms. There is no one "dyslexic" profile, no one standard set of characteristics. Instead, some students have speech articulation problems and halting verbal expression, while others speak fluently. Some experience eye-hand coordination immaturity, while others are able to assemble intricate puzzles and designs. Some seem to be in a world of their own, while others listen attentively and are very aware of social cues. Some cannot decode the simplest word, while others can read almost anything but have trouble comprehending what they read. Some reverse letters in reading and writing, whereas others do not.

There is also a great diversity regarding how strongly the dyslexic learning style occurs in individuals. Some people appear very similar to the typical learner in school. They may be a little delayed in learning to read and may experience some difficulty with spelling and grammar. Otherwise, they function very much like the rest of their peers. Other students can exhibit significant differences in many areas. They can be smaller physically and reach developmental milestones; for example, the loss of baby teeth at a much later age. They can have difficulty with most academic areas and seem unable to cope with social situations.

This great diversity of types and levels of dyslexia makes it very confusing for teachers to plan educational programs. There is no one standard curriculum for all people with this learning style; instead, each individual has to be assessed and a program carefully developed that will maximize success. Diagnostic tests can be helpful in beginning this process, but the teacher often learns about which techniques work best while working with the student.

The following are areas in which students with dyslexia can need individually designed intervention:

- ***Reading.*** Learners can have trouble with the decoding of words, fluent reading from left to right, and/or reading comprehension.
- ***Spelling.*** Even if word spellings are capably memorized over a short period of time, these word pictures often disappear from view. Homonyms and irregular words are particularly problematic.
- ***Phonemic Awareness.*** Students with dyslexia can have difficulty identifying sounds, knowing how many sounds there are, and knowing the order in which sounds occur in words. This weakness with phonemes, the smallest sounds in English, can affect reading, spelling, and the pronunciation of words.
- ***Auditory Discrimination.*** This inability to easily hear the small differences between sounds—especially vowel sounds—can have great impact on the acquisition of language skills.

- ***Handwriting.*** Eye-hand coordination immaturity and other problems can make it difficult for students to hold a pencil and to manipulate it with comfort and ease.
- ***Expository and Creative Writing.*** This can be an area of great fear and frustration. Problems with handwriting and spelling can make the act of writing cumbersome. Organizing thought into standard written English can also be hard.
- ***Math.*** Keeping track of where numbers are placed during computation problems can be difficult. Also, rote memorization tasks such as learning the multiplication tables can be a challenge.
- ***Visual-Motor Perception.*** This can affect two areas: the axis on which shapes can rotate, thus creating reversals in reading and writing, and the speed at which students can perform eye-hand coordination tasks.
- ***Gross Motor Coordination.*** Balance can be of particular concern. Individuals can be unaware of where their bodies are in space, and this can cause problems in the social arena when personal space is not recognized.
- ***Developmental Milestones.*** Some people with dyslexia seem to mature physically at a slower rate than the average population. Intellectual interests and ways of functioning socially can be more typical of students two or three years younger than of those of the same chronological age.
- ***ADD and ADHD*** (Attention Deficit Disorder and Attention Deficit Hyperactivity Disorder). ADD—or the inability to attend to outside stimuli, specifically the instruction of academics—can often occur in people with dyslexia. Physical hyperactivity, which also occurs in ADHD, is another common characteristic.
- ***Speech and Language.*** Problems can occur in articulation or in the fluent expression of grammatically correct English.
- ***Organization.*** Students can have trouble organizing both space and time. They can lose possessions and be unable to structure a large quantity of work into manageable units.
- ***Rote Memory Tasks.*** Words that have little meaning, such as the months of the year and phone numbers, are especially hard.
- ***Social and Behavioral.*** This difficulty can be the result of several factors. The child with dyslexia who is developmentally more like younger children will not be comfortable interacting with same-age peers. If the student is not being properly taught and is, instead, being embarrassed in front of peers, this sets up negative social situations. Last, some dyslexic people seem to need modeling and instruction in recognizing and responding appropriately to important social cues.
- ***Emotional.*** Most people with dyslexia have some sort of emotional struggle because, even if they are in nurturing homes and school settings, their educational experiences probably began with exposure to traditional curriculum and the resultant feelings of failure.

Eileen Simpson speaks of this in the preface of her book *Reversals*:

> There was something wrong with my brain. What had previously been a shadowy suspicion that hovered on the edge of consciousness became certain knowledge the year I was nine and entered fourth grade. I seemed to be like other children, but I was not like them. I could not learn to read or spell.*

WHAT CAUSES DYSLEXIA?

COMMON MYTHS

The most common myth, which is almost a stereotype because it is so widespread, is that all people with dyslexia reverse numbers and letters, and that this visual problem is the basis of the difficulty with academics. It is now known that people with dyslexia are as prone to reversals as anyone else, but not more so. In fact, children with typical learning styles commonly reverse letters and numbers until the age of seven. It is true that reversals can make written language confusing, but it is now commonly believed that the occurrence of reversals is neither a diagnostic sign nor a causal factor of dyslexia.

A second common myth is that people with dyslexia have impaired intelligence. In the past, IQ tests, which were largely based on language, were used to diagnose their needs. It is not surprising therefore, that they did not score well on these tests, because their problems are with language.

When an individual's needs are being assessed, it is critically important to find a diagnostician who is knowledgeable about how the dyslexic learning style affects test results. Then, true and helpful results can be obtained. It is now known that, most often, dyslexic people have average or above-average intelligence.

A third myth is that all people with dyslexia have ADD or ADHD. Although it is true that some do, this cannot be stated as a general rule.

A fourth myth, which is so very prevalent that it *is* a stereotype, is that gender is a factor, and that there are more males with dyslexia than females. Recent analyses have indicated, however, that this belief was based on studies that looked only at children who were already referred for services. New studies, which are examining large groups of children in school districts, are finding the same percentage of reading problems in girls as in boys. Many educators now believe that former studies are flawed because boys are more likely to be referred as a result of behavioral problems. It is also possible that some people still have higher academic expectations for boys than for girls.

---

*From *Reversals: A Personal Account of Victory over Dylexia* by Eileen Simpson (Houghton Mifflin Company, 1979). Used by permission.

As we turn to look at causes of dyslexia, therefore, many factors have been ruled out: It doesn't seem to be based on purely visual issues, on intelligence, on attention and behavior, or on gender. As educators, however, we commonly see students who seem so bright but who exhibit a wide range of symptoms—so what is causing their problems?

WHAT CURRENT RESEARCH IS SHOWING

Educators and researchers have been examining the issue of phonological processing, also called *phonemic awareness*. This is the knowledge of the sounds connected with written language and the ability to manipulate them so that words and sentences can be created. It appears to be a common area of difficulty for people with dyslexia; they have trouble remembering the sounds of letters. Even if they know all the letters and sounds in a given word, they have difficulty putting them together in the correct order. Blending sounds is hard. Is it any wonder, then, that reading and other language-based tasks are difficult?

At this point in time, it is commonly believed that difficulty with phonemic awareness is a root cause of the reading, writing, and spelling difficulties. It is often noticed that children with dyslexia have had trouble focusing on basic language tasks, such as rhyming words, which seems to come naturally to children who have a more typical learning style. For students with dyslexia to be able to readily associate the sounds with letters, they seem to need carefully structured, extensive, multisensory instruction.

It's fine to say that lack of phonemic awareness is a common area of concern, but what causes this difficulty with isolating, identifying, and manipulating sounds? The development of such new technology as Magnetic Resonance Imaging (MRI) is giving researchers many new tools to search for the basic cause of dyslexia. It is now generally believed that physiological differences in brain organization and structure are at the root of the dilemma. Something is different in the way the brain processes languages, and researchers are working hard to find out what that is.

Fascinating work is now being led by Dr. Sally E. Shaywitz, a pediatrician and researcher at the Yale School of Medicine. Her research team uses functional MRI to see the brain in action—to observe the brains of people who are actually thinking and reading. While people are reading, rapid successive images of their brains are being recorded on a computer screen. The areas of the brain that are more active show up as brighter images because the blood is carrying more oxygen to those parts. Since it is now known where reading processes such as sounding out words and comprehending print occur, it is possible to map what is happening while people read.

According to a March 1, 1998, article in the *Hartford Courant* by Robert A. Frahm and Rick Green, in their most current work the Shaywitz team studied both typical readers and people identified as having dyslexia. Subjects were asked to perform such tasks as silently reading pairs of nonsense words and pressing a button for "yes" or "no" to say whether the words rhymed, while their brains were being imaged on a computer screen. The researchers discovered that the brains of people with dyslexia showed less activity in the area of phonemic awareness.

Researchers at Stanford University, however, have concluded that brain activity in the visual portion of the brain may be highly influential. A December 9, 1997, article in the *Hartford Courant* by Michelle Guido, Knight Ridder newspapers, reports that there was less brain activity in the visual portions of the brains of five students with dyslexia than in the brains of five students with more typical learning styles. David Heeger, assistant professor of psychology and neuroscience and the head of the Stanford research team, cautions that just thinking of dyslexia as an issue with the language center of the brain may not be the whole answer. There may be other factors that we have not yet discovered.

What, therefore, does research show us about the root cause of dyslexia? It is probably safe to say that most people now agree that there is a physiological basis for the condition. It looks probable that the language center of the brain is involved, but there may be other important physiological factors. Research will continue, and more truths will most likely emerge in time. It is important to discover the root cause or causes, because this has significant implications for educational methodology.

WHAT DO LEARNING STYLES AND MULTIPLE INTELLIGENCES HAVE TO DO WITH DYSLEXIA?

It is well understood at this time that people learn in different ways, and that we all tend to have relative strengths and weaknesses in obtaining and processing information. The primary ways that we learn are as follows:

- ***Auditory.*** Knowledge is gained and remembered through the sense of hearing.
- ***Visual.*** Knowledge is gained and remembered through the sense of sight.
- ***Tactile-Kinesthetic.*** Knowledge is gained and remembered through the sense of touch and body movement.
- ***Analytic, or Left-Brained.*** Knowledge is best gained and understood when individual facts are presented in orderly, sequential ways.
- ***Global, or Right-Brained.*** Knowledge is best gained when a general principle is presented, from which facts can be understood.

These ways of obtaining information are not exclusive. In other words, it would be a rare person, indeed, who used only one of the above modalities and approaches to learn. Every person, however, does have a pattern of typical ways through which she or he obtains and processes information, and this is called that person's learning style. Everyone learns fastest and most readily when this important individual style is considered in planning and presenting academics.

In his book *Frames of Mind, the Theory of Multiple Intelligences* (Basic Books, 1993) Howard Gardner presents a theory by which he identifies seven different types of intelligence. Each of these intelligences is associated with a well-defined learning style. They are:

- ***Linguistic.*** People with this type of intelligence are good with, or excel at, language and easily learn to read and write with traditional curriculum.
- ***Logical-Mathematical.*** Learners with this kind of intelligence enjoy figuring things out and discovering patterns in groups of data. They do well in science and math.
- ***Spatial.*** These learners like to look at things and are skilled at assessing spatial relationships. They can become fine artists.
- ***Bodily-Kinesthetic.*** People with this kind of intelligence often enjoy and excel with movement. They often learn best when they are presented with hands-on activities.
- ***Musical.*** These people understand and respond to rhythms and tunes. Music can be used to help them remember facts and ideas.
- ***Interpersonal.*** This form of intelligence fosters good social abilities and understanding.
- ***Intrapersonal.*** People with a good amount of this intelligence understand themselves and their own needs very well.

As with the various ways of obtaining and processing information, these intelligences are not mutually exclusive. People do, however, have their own patterns, and they tend to rely on some forms of intelligences more than others. Students with dyslexia tend to have relative personal weaknesses in their linguistic intelligence; this often causes them to fail with traditional curriculum. They can, however, have many strengths in their other types of intelligences, and these should be noted and used as educational programs are presented.

THE STRENGTHS ASSOCIATED WITH DYSLEXIA

Most teachers who have worked with students with this learning style quickly realize that they are privileged to be with students who have amazing talents. They can have uncanny abilities to fix mechanical things. In a small private school, one student was known for his incredible ability to locate objects. If anyone lost something, often the first words spoken were, "Go ask Pedro. He'll know where it is." And he usually did. A short list of specific characteristics often seen is as follows:

- Curiosity
- Willingness to ask questions
- Ability to look at things differently, otherwise known as creative thinking
- Good sense of humor
- Lots of energy
- Lots of drive and ambition
- Willingness to work hard
- Good mechanical abilities
- Good spatial abilities
- Good artistic abilities
- Good musical abilities
- Ability to focus for a very long time on a task that interests them
- Ability to recognize patterns in a group of seemingly unrelated data
- Ability to understand concepts

When we think about Gardner's concept of multiple intelligence, the so-called dyslexic learning style makes a lot more sense. These students appear to have relative weaknesses in some areas of linguistic intelligence, but researchers are coming to believe that this is primarily in the area of phonemic awareness. It appears that whatever causes this particular weakness also causes significant strengths in other areas of intelligence. For example, spatial intelligence is good, and that is why many students with this learning style can fix just about anything. Also, logical-mathematical intelligence can be excellent, and patterns can easily be seen.

It is interesting to think about the concepts of right- and left-brain thinking, which have been discussed so much in recent years. When we look at this model, we see how the dyslexic learning style relies so much more on the right-brain, global thinking, than the left-brain analytic thinking. A researcher in neuroanatomy, Albert Galaburda, who has been studying the brains of people with dyslexia, has found that, whereas in typical learners the left hemisphere of the brain is larger than the right, people with dyslexia have symmetrical hemispheres. The two sides of the brain also communicate differently than do asymmetrical hemispheres. This can account for the unusual weaknesses and strengths associated with this learning style.

In the Mind's Eye: Visual Thinkers, Gifted People with Dyslexia and Other Learning Difficulties, Computer Images and the Ironies of Creativity by Thomas G. West (Prometheus Books, 1997) is a fascinating book.* According to West, the research shows that dyslexia is neurologically based and that differences in brain function cre-

---

*From Thomas G. West, *In the Mind's Eye* (Amherst, NY: Prometheus Books), Copyright 1997. Reprinted by permission of the publisher.

ate a wide variety of characteristics. This wide variety of characteristics is in itself a very important pattern. He states, "In the end, it may be that the most important and salient characteristic of the pattern is that each creative person is substantially different from the norm, the ordinary, but is also substantially different from other creative persons as well."

West also points out that the advantage of having a particular learning style is culture-based. A learning style that may be advantageous in one society may not be so in another. For example, in hunting-and-gathering cultures, people must have a good sense of direction and be alert and attuned to the variations in the natural world. Problems and challenges need to be creatively addressed. Reading and writing are not that important to survival.

I was recently in a university setting, where I had to find a person named Jeanette in a distant office. Because I got lost, she had to come and personally escort me to our destination. Jeanette commented, "I've noticed that writers tend to get lost when they're trying to find my office. They walk around, not noticing where they're going. It's odd." Linguistically gifted, but directionally challenged? Of course, not all writers are afflicted with this difficulty, but Jeanette did notice it as a common characteristic.

To summarize, West believes that people with the dyslexic learning style could have an advantage in hunting-and-gathering cultures, but in our current language-based culture, they suffer much trying to fit in. West further contends, however, that our society is changing—that with the advent of computers, we are being overrun with information, and people in business and other areas are struggling to deal with it. What is needed is an ability to see patterns in seemingly unrelated data, a creative way of approaching things, the energy and drive and ability to focus on a task long enough to solve a problem. According to West, in our future society, it may be the people with dyslexia who make significant contributions.

We must teach students with dyslexia well and have great respect for their abilities. They may be our leaders in future times.

FAMOUS PEOPLE WITH DYSLEXIA

A great many individuals with dyslexia have already contributed significantly to our society: Albert Einstein, Winston Churchill, Charles Darwin, Galileo, and Leonardo da Vinci. Most of these people, of course, were not labeled as having dyslexia, because the term wasn't in use until the late 1800s. Also, it is only in recent years that we have a good operational definition, one that helps us recognize the learning style. As we look at those well-known individuals, however, recorded information about them causes us to postulate that they were indeed blessed with this special way of looking at the world.

We will look in more depth into the history of Albert Einstein, using information from *In the Mind's Eye*. I am grateful to Thomas West for presenting such a compelling and fascinating story of Albert Einstein's early life.

Albert Einstein's early development as a child was very slow, and he had particular difficulty with language. His sister has written that, in his early years, members of his family were afraid that he would never learn to talk. In a letter, Einstein states the following about his early schooling, "As a pupil I was neither particularly good nor bad. My principal weakness was a poor memory and especially a poor memory for words and text. Only in mathematics and physics was I, through self study, far beyond the school curriculum, and also with regard to philosophy." One of his teachers, an instructor of Greek, told him, "You will never amount to anything."

Einstein had a lot of musical talent, but he was very disorganized. He had difficulties with spelling and a lack of interest in learning facts. And in mathematics? Apparently, he consistently had trouble with mathematical calculations. When he was seven years old, he was known to get his knuckles rapped for not being able to give quick, rote answers to questions of multiplication facts. He knew how to solve problems, but he made lots of errors with the details.

Einstein's family moved from Germany to Italy when he was fifteen years old. The original plan was for him to stay in the German high school and finish. But, in his own words, "I was summoned by my homeroom teacher who expressed the wish that I leave the school. To my remark that I had done nothing amiss, he replied only, 'Your mere presence spoils the respect of the class for me.' "

I myself, to be sure, wanted to leave school and follow my parents to Italy. But the main reason for me was the dull, mechanized method of teaching. Because of my poor memory for words, this presented me with great difficulties that it seemed senseless for me to overcome. I preferred, therefore, to endure all sorts of punishments, rather than learn to gabble by rote."

Einstein was certainly not a star pupil in the traditional schools of his day. He did manage to get a university education, studying physics instead of mathematics. When asked about this, he answered that he had a stronger intuition in physics—that he was able to better see the important patterns in the midst of the many distracting facts.

When he graduated, however, he was not able to find a teaching job. Unfortunately, many of his professors felt that he was intellectually arrogant, and they did not recommend him for teaching positions. Einstein expresses his despair at this time: "After all, I am nothing but a burden to my family. . . . It would indeed be better if I were not alive at all. Only the thought that I have always done whatever lay within my modest powers, and that year in, year out I do not permit myself a single pleasure, a distraction save that which my studies offer me, sustains me and must sometimes protect me from despair."

How fortunate for our culture that Einstein had the perseverance to continue. How fortunate, also, that in 1902, a good friend of his helped him get a job in a patent office. Einstein used his free time to formulate papers and published them three years later. Once the world saw his work, he was recognized as the genius he was.

Many more famous individuals, including Michael Farraday, George Patton, and Lewis Carroll, are profiled in *In the Mind's Eye*.This book is highly recommended as a source of excellent information about famous people with dyslexia.

A HISTORICAL PERSPECTIVE

The term *dyslexia* has been used since the late 1880s. It has, however, been mostly a medical term, with educators preferring the label "learning disabled." However, "dyslexia" is now also becoming a recognized term in educational circles. Most people understand it as a subtype of learning disability.

A major pioneer in the field was Dr. James Hinshelwood, an ophthalmologist in Scotland. Beginning in 1896, he was one of the first doctors to do clinical studies on children who couldn't read. He believed that what he called "congenital word blindness" was based on either brain defects or brain injury.

Dr. Samuel Orton, the American neurologist, was a major contributor to the field. Starting work in 1919, he believed that the reading problems he saw in intelligent children were based on neurological factors. He postulated that the hemispheres of the brains of children with these issues were equally dominant, and because of this, the children would see almost double, or mirror images. He speculated that language factors were also involved.

Dr. Orton's views on dyslexia were not widely accepted at the time. Psychoanalytic theory was popular, and educators believed that academic problems of seemingly bright people were based on emotional factors.

Dr. Orton teamed up with a psychologist and Research Associate named Anna Gillingham to create a multisensory learning program for people with dyslexia, but this approach was largely unknown in the wider culture. Mostly, private schools and individual tutors used the approach. It wasn't until the 1960s that dyslexia came to be an issue that was even discussed in the popular press. At that time, educators had widely divergent views, some even stating that dyslexia was an imaginary condition—that, in reality, it did not exist.

Fortunately, work on this perplexing condition has continued. We owe a great deal to the researchers who have continued to document characteristics of the learning style and who have never stopped looking for causes. They are now being helped by the new technology, which is greatly expanding their abilities to seek the truth.

We also owe a great deal to the educators, parents, and people with dyslexia themselves, who have continued to express the belief that the condition exists. They have sought help. They have refused to allow this learning style to go unnoticed. Their advocacy has created the climate for the advances of knowledge in the field.

INTERVIEW WITH HELEN

Helen is in her seventies. She has raised six children and now has several grandchildren. She lives on a beautiful farm in a rural area. She is very interested in botany and is an avid gardener.

When did you first hear about dyslexia?

I heard about dyslexia, although not named as such, when the son of my mother's friend was being tutored by my grandmother. She, the friend, read something about learning disabilities and then got her son to write something. He did it backward, and that was what she'd been reading about.

And my grandmother's way of teaching was helpful to her because she was very much the "you start at the beginning and so forth" type. That was the first time I knew there was such a thing as a learning disability, and I must have been thirteen. And no one ever told me that I had a learning disability.

I knew in college that I had trouble reading, compared with other people, and I'd known forever that I couldn't spell, and it didn't seem to be something that I could learn to do. And I can remember that when I was trying to learn to read, my father being furious with me, and saying "/k/, /k/, /k/, cat." And I'd start it with a "t."

And partly, I was taught; I went to a so-called progressive school in New York, and I was supposedly taught to read by sight recognition and not to sound out any words, so saying "/k/" to me, didn't mean anything.

When did you first think of yourself as having dyslexia?

The first time I associated dyslexia with myself was when my son, Peter, was diagnosed, and at that point, I was in my forties. I went to Dr. Smith in Boston, and Dr. Smith said, "Well, he has dyslexia."

And then he described it, and I said, "Oh, that fits me."

And he said, "Well, without a doubt, you passed it to your son." And it was kind of a relief to know that, indeed, there was a reason why I had problems.

Because, for instance, when I was in first grade, I remember taking a list of spelling words to a test, and I remember being caught with my list. And the teacher kept me after the others went out to play and, you know, I was in tears and she said, "Well, you'll never do that again," and I said, "No, I'll never do that," but I sort of felt, "I'm a cheat. Basically, at heart, I'm a cheat."

And at a workshop, many years later, which had nothing to do with language but had to do with remembering, I suddenly thought, you know, I recognized that I had a problem and I thought of a solution for it, and for that, I've labeled myself a cheat all my life—and it really was quite sensible of me. But it took a lot of having raised a child who was dyslexic and who got treated for it and all that sort of thing before I reached that point.

Has it been difficult for you to have dyslexia?

The disadvantages of not being able to spell are tremendous. In college, I would sit in an exam and try to think how to spell something and then, having failed that, I'd try to think of a word I could substitute. That slows you down. And I still have that trouble.

Does having dyslexia still affect you?

I don't like to write letters; I never write letters. And I thought, you know, I can overcome this, I'm a big girl now. And I sat down the other day not too long ago and started to write a letter, and I hadn't gotten more than a sentence and a half down before I thought, I don't know how to spell. And I don't want to write with a misspelling. I mean, to my children, I don't mind if I misspell, but to somebody else, I guess I still am defensive about that.

My husband's son is dyslexic, and much more so than either my son or me, and he had a terrible, terrible time learning to read. He was tutored every single day for years. And now, if he needs to read something, he can do it. He can find something in a book and look it up. But if he has to fix something, he always tries first to do it on his own. He's very good at fixing things, because he doesn't read the instructions. He sees how it works, puts it together as if it's a puzzle. He would rather do it that way. If he's desperate, he will go and look something up, but he's the biggest fixer. I'm not a good fixer, but that's because I've never really tried to be.

I have a funny story about my son's and my dyslexia. The funny story I have is that there was a program—it was an actual trial on television. It was one of the first televised trials, and Peter and I watched it, and we were fascinated by it, and we were into all the different aspects of the case. The rest of the family was in and out. At the end of this, neither Peter nor I could name a single person in the trial, and everyone else in the family knew all the names. And he and I knew all the concepts. And it was just amazing to us. And we laughed about it, because that was just the epitome of it. We both had the concepts.

And you were the ones interested in it.

Yes. And Peter said once, when he was still in high school, "You know, William (his brother) reads awfully fast, but I remember some of the things better than he does of what we've read." And so, I think he has compensated. It's very hard when you have a speed reader around to feel good about yourself.

Do you have any other memories of how having dyslexia affected you when you were young?

I can remember my father spanking me because I didn't read "tra-la-la-la" in Mother Goose. I could find you the poem in Mother Goose to this day. Now, part of that was a struggle between us, because I know that I could have memorized "tra-la-la," or whatever it was in the time that we spent on it. What I couldn't do was see the difference between "tra" and "la" because they're both this way and a little thing following, and since I hadn't had anything that said "t" has one sound and "l" has another, it was asking more than I could do. And he felt so bad about spanking me. And I never felt bad about it, because I knew it was coming. I was infuriating him and so when it finally happened, it was not a surprise to me, nor did he hurt me in any great way.

But it wasn't until years afterward that I thought, oh, you know, it wasn't just that I was trying to infuriate him. That was there, too, I think, but it was that I really did have this problem, and that's what was frustrating him; he couldn't get it across to me.

He couldn't help you.

Yeah, he was saying "/t/, /t/, /t/." I could see he was getting mad, so I was playing games, too. So it was not a case of child abuse at all. It was one of those things that happens between individuals.

CHAPTER 2

ASSESSMENT AND DIAGNOSIS

The area of testing and diagnosis can be intimidating because of the special vocabulary associated with it and because of the tendency of some diagnosticians to present large quantities of factual data. Identification of the student's main issues, needs, and strengths can get lost in this confusing mass. This chapter will attempt to cut through the confusion by clearly outlining the important aspects of a good evaluation.

WHAT ASSESSMENTS CAN SHOW

Standardized tests offer one type of assessment instrument. Good observation, curriculum based assessment, and informal measures can also provide valuable information. The following are the main areas in which to look for factors that may be inhibiting a student's learning.

- ***Medical.*** It is first important to find out if a student has any physical impairments. Hearing and vision tests can be done, as well as screenings for epilepsy and other ailments.
- ***Intellectual.*** In this area, we look at the student's cognitive ability.
- ***Educational.*** Here, we look at where the student is currently functioning in specific academic areas such as reading, spelling, and math.
- ***Emotional.*** Tests called projective tests are often administered to gain insight into a student's psychological makeup.
- ***Social.*** At times, interviews to assess a student's behavioral strategies are conducted.
- ***Speech and Language.*** Here, we look at specific areas of language functioning, such as word retrieval and vocabulary.
- ***Gross-motor and Fine-motor Skills.*** A student's ability to function in the physical world is assessed. Factors such as balance and eye-hand coordination are examined.

- ***Neurological.*** This evaluation is usually conducted after other areas have been explored. Here, a student's central nervous system, including the brain, is examined.
- ***Home Study.*** Interviews can be conducted to focus on how the student's wider culture is impacting her performance at school. For example, it is very important to discover parents' and other caregivers' feelings about the student's schooling. Are language factors influential: Is the student, in fact, speaking a language other than English at home or in the community?

WHO DOES THE ASSESSMENTS?

Medical doctors examine a student's physical structure and functioning; school nurses can assist. It can be important, however, to find a specialist in an area such as vision if there is a suspicion that there may be a problem in this area. A person can have excellent visual acuity, which is what a general screening measures, but have trouble with eye-tracking, the ability to comfortably move the eyes from left to right and from the end of one line down to another. That same person can also have difficulty focusing on print for an extended period of time.

The important thing to remember is to keep looking if something seems suspicious. If the doctor thinks that something is a little odd but is not clear about what is happening, ask her or him to consult with a specialist in the area.

In most states, school psychologists give and evaluate the intelligence tests. Usually, the whole evaluation given by this professional is called a psychological evaluation and can include tests on many areas of functioning, such as emotional, behavioral, fine-motor, and others. In some states, an educational diagnostician does both intelligence and educational testing.

Special education teachers usually administer the educational tests. Occasionally, group standardized tests are at least referred to as the student's academic functioning is being examined. Also, very valuable information can be gained from direct observation of the student in the classroom and from an examination of her work. The classroom teacher plays a pivotal role in this.

School psychologists are often responsible for the assessment of the student's emotional needs as well as the behavioral strategies. At times, social workers and psychiatrists can be involved with this as well. Independent therapists, with permission from parents, can provide input.

Speech and language clinicians conduct the speech and language testing. Occupational and/or physical therapists usually assess a student's fine-motor and gross-motor skills. Neurologists—sometimes at special clinics—look at a student's neurological makeup. Social workers or school psychologists usually do home studies.

WHAT ARE THE MAIN TESTS?

Tests are considered standardized when they are given to a large group and typical response patterns or "standards" are established. When this happens, the test is said to have norms. Individual student response patterns are then compared to these norms. The following tests are frequently administered to gain information about a student's learning style:

WECHSLER INTELLIGENCE SCALE FOR CHILDREN—III (WISC—III)

This is the most frequently used diagnostic instrument for assessing intelligence. It is appropriate for children from six to sixteen years. Before six, the Wechsler Preschool and Primary Scale of Intelligence—R (WPPSI—R) is used, and the Wechsler Adult Intelligence Scale—Revised (WAIS—R) is used for older teenagers and adults. Both of these tests are based on the same concepts as those of the WISC and are adapted because of developmental issues.

The WISC is comprised of twelve subtests, each of which tends to measure a specific ability. For example, abstract thinking is assessed in the subtest Similarities, in which students are asked to tell what is the same about pairs, such as "a lamp" and "the sun." Eye-hand coordination is measured in the subtest Coding, in which students are asked to quickly write down symbols that are associated with numbers on a preexisting form. Standard scores are calculated for each of these subtests. Standard scores range from 0–20, with 9–11 being average scores.

The WISC subtests are divided into two types: Verbal and Performance. The former focuses more on language-based skills, whereas the latter taps visual-motor abilities. By analyzing a student's performance on each, it is possible to gain a picture of relative strengths and weaknesses.

The WISC gives us three intelligence quotients (IQ): A Verbal IQ, a Performance IQ, and a resultant Full-Scale IQ. The theoretical IQ range is from 0–200. "Average" is considered to be from 80 to 120.

For students with dyslexia, IQ scores can be very misleading. First of all, students with dyslexia have language issues. They therefore often perform poorly on the language-based subtests—especially on the ones that have little meaning, such as Digit Span, which asks a student simply to repeat series of numbers. This subtest is based on rote, short-term auditory memory, a classic weakness for people with dyslexia. Also, some people with dyslexia have weaknesses on some of their visual motor skills, so it is an oversimplification to say the dyslexia can be diagnosed by a discrepancy between a low Verbal IQ and a high Performance IQ. Some students have issues in both areas, which lowers both the Verbal and Performance IQs.

In general, many people with dyslexia have weaknesses on the following subtests on the WISC:

- Information, in which they are asked to recall and restate factual information about the world.
- Arithmetic, in which they are asked to solve word problems and do mathematical calculations in their heads.
- Digit Span, in which they are asked to repeat series of numbers.
- Coding, in which they are asked to quickly copy geometric shapes in a code format.

Difficulty with these subtests and others can artificially lower IQ scores. Therefore, most people with dyslexia, in fact, have higher intellectual potential than is measured by the Full-Scale IQ on the WISC. It is also important to remember that the main pattern of the dyslexic learning style is diversity. People have all types of strengths and weaknesses that can have an impact on test performance. When a student is suspected of having dyslexia, therefore, it is critically important for the school psychologist who is administering and evaluating the test to have an understanding of the learning style.

Generally, what shows up on testing is what shows up in the classroom: A student with dyslexia has many surprising strengths and many surprising weaknesses. This wide scatter, and the great discrepancies, may be the most important diagnostic sign.

Woodcock-Johnson Psycho-Educational Battery—Revised—Cognitive Scale

A second main test for assessing intellectual potential and learning is the Woodcock-Johnson Psycho-Educational Battery—Revised—Cognitive Scale (WJR). This test is gaining popularity among psychologists who do a lot of testing of students with dyslexia. Dr. Peter B. Martin, a licensed psychologist who is in private practice in Northfield, Massachusetts, prefers this test over the WISC. In speaking of the WJR, he states, "It is only one of two tests in the field (the other being the Kaufman Adolescent and Adult Intelligence Test) constructed on the Horn-Cattell model, and the Horn-Cattell model is the only empirically supported model that we have. Horn-Cattell is like Gardner in that it's a theory of individual intelligences. It breaks up intelligence into much smaller units than Gardner. For example, kinesthetic intelligence is probably made up of several Horn-Cattell intelligences.

The Woodcock-Johnson gives you a profile of abilities, with relative strengths and weaknesses. The achievement tests (the Woodcock-Johnson Psycho-Educational Battery) were constructed and normed at the same time as the cognitive measures; this allows direct comparison of scores. You not only get for a single student a comprehensive profile of cognitive abilities, but you also get a comprehensive profile of academic achievement.

You can look at clusters to see where there are patterns of cognitive abilities that predict academic skills. For example, for reading, a person needs good abilities in auditory processing, processing speed, vocabulary, and short-term memory. These four abilities predict reading better than an entire IQ battery. Therefore, this is the most powerful approach to detecting aptitude and achievement discrepancies; that is, learning disabilities.

Woodcock-Johnson Psycho-Educational Battery—Revised: Tests of Achievement

Achievement tests fall in the educational assessment area and measure at what level a student is currently functioning in well-defined academic areas, as compared with her peers. One frequently used test is the Woodcock-Johnson Psycho-Educational Battery—Revised: Tests of Achievement. This test is administered individually and has subtests that fall into the general areas of reading, math, written language, and knowledge. Two examples of subtests in the written language area are Writing Sample and Writing Fluency. The former asks a student to write very specific words and sentences, responding to pictures and direct instructions. The latter adds the element of time, asking students to respond to given pictures and to write as many sentences as they can in a given time period.

Wide Range Achievement Test

Another frequently administered achievement test is the Wide Range Achievement Test (WRAT). There are three subtests: Spelling, Reading, and Arithmetic. As with all tests, it is important to know what students are asked to do in order to gain a real sense of what the test scores mean. For the WRAT Spelling, students are simply asked to write down some dictated words. They complete mathematical computation problems for the Arithmetic, and decode presented words for the Reading. No reading comprehension is involved.

Additional Achievement Tests

Other frequently used achievement tests are the Peabody Individual Achievement Test—Revised and the Key Math test. The Lindamood Auditory Conceptualization Test (LAC) taps auditory discrimination and is, therefore, an important test to diagnose phonological awareness issues.

The Peabody Picture Vocabulary Test is an interesting assessment instrument, especially for students with dyslexia. On this test, four pictures are presented on a given page. Students are told a word and asked to point to the picture that best represents that word. This test can sometimes show surprisingly good results for a person with dyslexia who has some language and other issues but has a good vocabulary.

Because an IQ score can be obtained from the Peabody Picture Vocabulary Test, this good score can often be yet another indication that a low IQ on another test may be due to issues not related to intellectual potential.

School psychologists will sometimes administer the Bender-Gestalt. Here, students are asked to copy geometric and other shapes onto a piece of paper. Visual-motor issues as well as emotional problems can be seen on this test.

A very common test for looking at a person's emotional life is the Thematic Apperception Test. Here, a psychologist chooses from a group of pictures and shows them, one by one, to a student. The student is asked to make up a story. The psychologist writes the story down and evaluates it later for clues to emotional needs and strengths.

WHAT DO SOME OF THESE TESTING TERMS MEAN?

- ***Screening Tests.*** These give a quick picture of a person's ability in a given area. Sometimes they are used to figure out where more extensive testing should occur.
- ***Diagnostic Tests.*** These are usually administered individually and show a much more in-depth picture. You can gain real insight into a person's learning style from these tests.
- ***Norm-referenced Tests.*** Most diagnostic tests are norm referenced. That means that a large number of people have taken the test after it was initially created, and their performances have been recorded. Statistics have been developed indicating a typical response for a given age or grade. When an individual student now takes the test, her performance is compared and evaluated by using these statistics.
- ***Criterion-referenced Tests.*** These tests are less common. They measure a person's performance against a specific standard, such as how many multiplication facts the student knows.
- ***Raw Score on a Test.*** This is the number of points a person earns on a given test. Usually, the raw score has no innate meaning and must be understood in terms of the statistics for the given test.
- ***Age Level Test Score.*** This score indicates that the person has performed at the same level as the average person of a given age.
- ***Grade Level Test Score.*** This score indicates that a person has performed at the same level as the average person in a given grade. Often, these scores are reported in terms of years and months. For example, 3.6 means the sixth month of third grade.

- ***Percentile Test Scores.*** This score shows the relative performance of an individual compared with students of either the same age or the same grade. If, for example, a student earns a percentile of 83, that means that she performed at the same level as or better than 83 out of 100 people of her age or grade.
- ***Standard Test Scores.*** These scores are derived from raw scores and reflect how far below or above average the student is performing in a given area. For example, on the WISC, standard scores range from 0 to 20, with ten being an average score. If a student earns a standard score of 14 on Vocabulary, for example, that indicates that she is functioning well above average.

THE CULTURAL BIAS OF TESTS

It is generally recognized at this time that all tests are culturally biased. Even tests that seemingly have no language requirements are influenced by culture. For example, if a young child is asked to copy a geometric shape with a pencil, her performance will be influenced by whether or not she was exposed to writing implements at home and in her community. If she has rarely held a pencil or crayon, this will affect her ability to copy.

Does this young child feel comfortable with a person who is not from her culture? What has her family taught her about relating to strangers? Should she be outgoing and talkative, or has she been taught that the appropriate role of a child is to be withdrawn and very quiet?

The overt cultural biases of standardized tests are easily seen. They often present pictures based on a set of images that are common in one place and not another. The vocabulary which is used will be distinct to a particular group. In the extreme case, the student being tested will not be fluent with the language of the test.

Should we, therefore, not test students who do not come from the primary culture? Research is showing us that there are no innate differences in abilities between people from different cultures, and that dyslexia occurs in all cultures and languages. Therefore, we will do a real disservice to some students if we allow the limitations of our current tests to keep us from trying to diagnose their needs. The tests do show a picture of a person's current functioning. If much care is taken to understand and make adjustments for cultural differences, they can begin the process of helping students from different cultures. The key is to be sensitive and alert. The following will help assure a more accurate assessment:

- Testing should be done in the primary language or dialect, if possible.
- Great care should be spent in establishing rapport.
- A comfortable and safe testing room should be provided.
- Evaluators should supplement the testing with interviews to gain more information about the student's home life and community.

WHAT TESTS CAN'T DO—LIMITATIONS

Tests are not the final answer. They are merely a picture of a person's functioning on a given day at a given time. Even though they attempt to gain information about a person's innate abilities, this is often impossible because of intervening variables such as behavioral issues, emotional issues, and cultural factors.

A main concern about testing—especially for people with dyslexia—is that the IQ score is usually affected by weakness in the learning style. This is especially true for students who have difficulties in both language and visual-motor areas because both the Verbal and Performance IQs are depressed. Even though school psychologists will often state this during team meetings and write this in their reports, some people just focus on the number. In our culture, IQ scores have a lot of potency, and a student can be misperceived as having a lower potential because of them. For this reason, some psychologists try to avoid giving IQ scores for people with dyslexia.

Tests are the starting place as we try to plan an effective program. If their limitations are understood, they can at least point us in the right direction to begin work.

SPECIFIC DIAGNOSTIC SIGNS OF DYSLEXIA

The most important diagnostic signpost of this fascinating learning style is diversity. Therefore, students show a wide range of issues and strengths. The main diagnostic sign, therefore, is surprising strengths and surprising weaknesses. There is a wide scatter among test results, and an especially wide discrepancy between academic performance—often reading—and perceived ability.

The following specific signs are commonly found:

- Wide disparity between listening comprehension of text and reading comprehension.
- Greater ability to decode real words than nonsense words.
- Slow and painful reading.
- Many decoding errors, especially with the order of letters.
- Ongoing difficulty with decoding, even when reading comprehension is improving.
- Weakness in spelling, which can be even greater than the weakness in reading.
- Wide disparity between functioning in math and reading. In some cases, people with dyslexia also have problems with math because of difficulty with computation. But there are also some students with dyslexia who are very talented mathematicians.

WHAT THE LABEL *DYSLEXIA* CAN AND CANNOT DO

The term *dyslexia* has been in use since the late 1800s but has never been a political or legal term. In the 1950s and 1960s, it was required that students be labeled in a special needs category in order to receive special education services. As students with dyslexia weren't emotionally, mentally, or physically handicapped, they didn't fit into any of the existing categories; therefore, they often were not given help.

The term *learning disabilities* was introduced in 1963 at a national conference. Finally, a label was created that could qualify students for services. At this time, it is estimated that students with learning disabilities make up approximately half of the ten percent of students receiving special education. Most professionals believe that at least half of this five percent have dyslexia.

A second advantage of being labeled as learning disabled is that modifications can then be made in standardized testing situations, such as allowing time-and-a-half or untimed tests. This can be helpful, especially for students trying to get into college. Some colleges also allow modifications in their language requirements for students with dyslexia.

The label, therefore, qualifies students for appropriate services and modifications; it is also, however, extremely limited. It cannot delineate the strengths of a person, or of her motivation or her willingness to work hard. It gives no sense of the person—is she depressed, or is she happily pursuing creative work outside of school? The label tells us only where to start to look for appropriate instructional methods and programs; it is only a beginning.

WHAT CAN THE CLASSROOM TEACHER DO?

In a word: a *lot*. Teachers are in a unique position because they spend a great deal of time with the student. They see her in a wide variety of academic and social situations. They can provide very important information about the student's personality style, social skills, behavior during stress, and behavior when she is succeeding. They can point out areas of strength that may not be evident during formal evaluation. They can be strong advocates to make sure that the student receives the effective help that she deserves.

TIPS FOR TEACHERS AND PARENTS

- If evaluators are speaking in jargon, ask them to explain the terms they are using. Do not be embarrassed to do this. They need to speak in simple language.

- If you do not understand what a test score means, ask the evaluator to show you the test task, or to give you an example of it. For example, if the school psychologist reports that the student performed well on the Block Design subtest of the WISC III, ask what the student specifically had to do to earn such a good score.
- Remember that no matter how skilled a tester is you are fortunate to have had plenty of time with the student. An evaluator is often a stranger and, at best, has only a few hours with the student. You can contribute greatly to the understanding of what the test data mean.
- Remember that teachers and parents can become skilled observers and can contribute a great deal to an assessment of a student's learning style. Standardized tests are not necessarily better; they are just faster.
- Providing samples of the student's work, both from the classroom and from home, can be very valuable.
- If you don't understand something that is reported by an evaluator, keep asking questions until you do.
- See the evaluation as a team effort, not as one or two specialists coming in and providing all the answers.
- Remember that postevaluation conferences, apart from the team meeting, are available to parents.
- Be aware of how the student is reacting to the evaluation situation. If she seems upset, talk with the evaluators about this. Testing should be a positive, healing experience.
- If a label is established and the student is made aware of this, be sure that she understands what the label means. A label of dyslexia means that she has an interesting learning style with some learning strengths and some learning weaknesses. She can do very well in school once she is taught by the proper methods, and this will be provided as soon as possible. She is smart and capable.

INTERVIEW WITH NAOMI

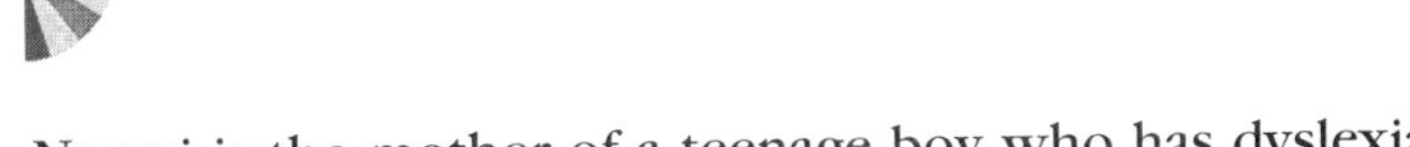

Naomi is the mother of a teenage boy who has dyslexia. Naomi works as a midwife. She also is now pursuing advanced studies.

What was the testing experience like for you?

It was the meetings after the testing. That's what I remember. One of the things they talked about was, the analogy was storing all your utensils in one drawer; so when you go to look for something—to retrieve something—they're all there, but they're not necessarily sorted or in order, so it takes longer to retrieve stuff. And considering that's how we store things in our drawers, I thought, that made sense to me. That was one way they described Malcolm's learning style.

There was another thing about organization in general, and there was some label for it, which I can't remember. But it's hard for Malcolm to track many things that are going on. And they made recommendations about what would help with that, many of which Ms. Thomas uses at school, in terms of keeping things organized and ordered.

But some of those recommendations in terms of our house are kind of difficult, so that was frustrating. It was sort of like, "Oh dear, we're going to have to find another house," which of course was not an option—just because it's not my organizational style.

So they were telling you to do something that you didn't feel you could follow through with at home?

It was pretty hard.

INTERVIEW WITH FRAN

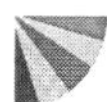

Fran, who has dyslexia herself, has raised three children with this learning style. She now works as an advocate for students who have difficulties with learning using traditional curriculum.

How did you first get interested in the whole area of dyslexia?

Well, before I had children, I was a social worker, so I like people. And when my oldest son was born, by the time he was about one and one-half, I began asking questions because he wasn't developing language, to the point where I had him tested to see if he had normal hearing. I kept asking questions and I kept going to experts and I kept getting all the wrong answers.

By the time he was in first grade, I finally took him down to Children's Hospital, and he was identified as having dyslexia. As they started to tell me about it, I realized that I had the same disorder. I kept saying, "Well, I do that. I do that."

Somebody told me that I was going to need to know about the law, and so I started taking any opportunity to learn about what disabilities there are, how you identify them, and what is the best practice as far as remediation is concerned. And from there, I went into the law. That's how I got started as an advocate. Subsequently, my two other children were also diagnosed with dyslexia.

When you said that, in the early years, you took your son to experts and they gave you the wrong answers, what do you mean by "the wrong answers"?

Initially, they told me that it was developmental, that he'd outgrow it, that it wasn't anything to be worried about. I was constantly told it was normal. Of course, that was 22 years ago. I now know, through one of the leading language people in the country, that you can actually identify dyslexia as early as six months.

Sometimes people are reluctant to have students tested because of the stigma of the label. What do you think about that?

I think it's crazy. Kids can sit there in kindergarten and know they're different from the child next to them. It's a whole lot easier to understand that you have a learning disorder—that there is a different way of teaching you and that you can learn—than that you're stupid.

I've seen children in the gifted category who can't read. And if you're sitting next to Johnny, who isn't as bright but can read, you think you're stupid.

Often, there are inconsistencies; one day you do better than another day, or if you're very bright, you cover up because you guess and you look at the pictures and you have a photographic memory, so you can hide a lot. But you still can't read and you can't write and you can't express yourself. You know, these students believe that they're stupid, and they're often told, "You're not motivated."

The WISC is terribly important, the intelligence test, because that scatter that you would normally find with a learning disability will give you indications of what's working and what's not. You can see whether you've got a verbal or a nonverbal disability.

You really need somebody who can take a good look, and there are wonderful things you can do to fix it. You don't have to just exist.

CHAPTER 3

ABOUT SPECIAL EDUCATION

THE LAW

In 1975, the United States Congress passed a critically important piece of legislation for people with dyslexia. This law is called the Education for All Handicapped Children Act (PL 94-142). It was updated in 1990 and renamed the Individuals with Disabilities Education Act (IDEA-PL 105-17). For the purposes of this law, dyslexia is considered a subtype of learning disabilities. This law requires the following for all students:

- A free and unbiased assessment
- Free appropriate education and special services to meet special needs
- Education in the least restrictive environment
- The opportunity for parents to be involved in the educational decision making for their children.

Under IDEA, the federal government gives states money to provide these special services. There are a number of requirements, defining both who is qualified to receive services and how these services must be provided. Most students with dyslexia, who are evaluated by a competent professional who is aware of this learning style, meet the criterion to receive services.

Two other laws are important to know about: Section 504 of the Rehabilitation Act of 1973 and the Americans with Disabilities Act of 1990. These civil rights laws are different from IDEA in two ways. First, they state that individuals should not be discriminated against because of any handicap (a learning difficulty is considered a handicap) throughout their lifetime, and that modifications should be made to meet individual needs. This therefore protects students with dyslexia as they enter college and the world of work. Second, the laws do not have the rigid qualifications for services upon which IDEA is based. This makes some people eligible for modifications who may have issues, such as organizational issues, that affect their lives but do not necessarily qualify them for the label "learning disabled."

The types of modifications that Section 504 requires are often simple and inexpensive. They can include things like the following:

- Teaching through multisensory instruction
- Not lowering grades because of poor spelling
- Letting students take some tests orally
- Helping students create and maintain a homework journal
- Providing in-service training for teachers and parents to help them understand special needs

These modifications are, in effect, common sense adaptations. They can, however, be critically important in helping students with dyslexia to be successful.

REFERRAL

Schools have developed systems through which students are enabled to receive special services. These systems usually contain the following elements:

- Referral
- Formal evaluation
- The team meeting
- Development of the Individual Educational Plan (IEP)
- The annual review
- The three-year evaluation

We will first look at issues related to referral, as this begins the whole process. Here, classroom teachers, parents, and other teachers play a major role. Parents, for example, know about the development of a child prior to starting school. Did he, for example, have difficulty learning to speak? Is he starting to fight with his younger sister now that the school year has begun? Is he having trouble sleeping?

Classroom teachers are in a unique position to see the student's academic and social functioning. Is he having trouble learning the sounds of the letters? Does he never finish an assignment on time? Is he isolated and withdrawn on the playground during recess?

Other teachers can also play a key role. The physical education teacher can note if he is able to perform age-appropriate gross-motor movements. The art teacher can observe fine-motor skills. The music teacher can notice if he can stay focused on a page of sheet music while singing or playing an instrument, or if his eyes wander.

The most important thing is to notice what is happening with the child. For this purpose, use the following observation techniques:

- ***Relax.*** Take a few deep breaths and try to release from your mind any preconceptions of things you think you will observe.
- ***Give Yourself Uninterrupted Time for Your Observation.*** This may be difficult, especially if you are responsible for large groups of children. Consider asking another adult, such as a teacher's aide, to teach a mini-lesson to the whole group. Five minutes of well-focused time are worth much more than a half hour of distracted observation.
- ***Plan for Several Observation Sessions.*** In your first session, just freely observe the student and see what happens. Jot down notes of possible problem areas and plan for where and when you will observe next. For example, if you noticed that your student had trouble beginning silent reading, next observe during math and see if he is similarly distracted when beginning independent work. Continue observing in different settings and at different times, until you feel that you can come up with some hypotheses regarding the student's learning style.
- ***Write Down Your Hypotheses.*** Then, watch the student as much as you can to see if your hypotheses are correct. Write down specific examples of behaviors that point to difficulties with learning with traditional curriculum.
- ***Talk with Other Adults.*** Ask if they have observed the same or different behaviors in other settings and at other times.
- ***Check the Student's School Records.*** See if there is a recorded history of any unusual behaviors.

If you follow these steps, you will have a lot of information to bring to the referral process. Usually, when a student is officially referred, teachers are asked to fill out a form outlining the areas of concern. It you've spent the time in focused observation, it will be very easy for you to complete this form and to provide critically important information that will help direct future steps.

Sometimes, a principal asks classroom teachers and other professionals, such as special education teachers, to meet prior to initiating formal evaluation. This can be called a child study meeting, and it can be used for the purpose of determining if classroom or instructional modifications can be made that will allow the student to be successful without official special education intervention.

FORMAL EVALUATION

Some students with very mild dyslexia can succeed with minor classroom and instructional modifications. Most students with dyslexia , however, profit from going through formal evaluation. This not only qualifies them for a wide range of services but also provides valuable information on the type and amount of services required, and where these services should be provided.

Chapter 2, "Assessment and Diagnosis," deals in more depth with some of the concerns related to testing students with dyslexia. Here, let us look at some of the issues regarding the formal evaluation process.

Parents have to be notified in writing of the school's wish to test a child. Parents can either grant permission or refuse, and this refusal immediately stops the whole special education process. As it is often teachers who first speak with parents about the possible need for evaluation, let us first look at some questions parents ask about this big step:

➠ *"Will my child be singled out and made to feel different because of the testing?"*

The short answer is yes, students are always aware that something unusual is happening to them when they are being tested. They need opportunities to discuss their feelings about this and to be reassured that the testing is being done to help their teachers learn how to teach them most effectively. They must understand that there is nothing wrong with them, and the testing is definitely not being done to prove how badly they are doing in school. They are being tested because people care about them.

School psychologists, special education teachers, and other evaluators are usually very sensitive to the issue of the stigma of the testing. They often speak with the classroom teacher and try to form a plan that will create the least disruption for the child. Testing should be a positive experience, in which the student feels that he is important enough for his teachers to try to figure out how to best teach him.

➠ *"Will we understand all those fancy tests and numbers? We hear that this testing stuff can be very confusing."*

Poorly presented, evaluation data can do more to confuse than to enlighten. Tell parents that you are committed to understanding the results, yourself, and that you will be supportive of them if they need to ask questions about the evaluation. The evaluation is meant to serve their children's needs. Together, you will make sure that the evaluators keep explaining until the basic results are understood.

➠ *"What are the eligibility guidelines for special education?"*

To qualify for special services, it needs to be documented that the student has a basic issue in a process such as attention or expression and that he has a significant discrepancy between potential and achievement in one of the academic areas. His educational performance needs to be affected, as evidenced by poor grades, and the degree of severity of his learning difficulty must require special services, not just classroom modifications. His learning issues cannot be caused by environmental factors or such other factors as nonattendance at school.

➠ *"But won't my child feel horrible about himself if he is labeled as learning disabled?"*

This issue certainly needs to be addressed. Once again, the student needs many opportunities to discuss his feelings, ideally both at home and at school. Some specific suggestions for helping students with this are offered in Chapter 16 in this resource: "Self-Esteem and Other Emotional Needs."

If the student truly has dyslexia, he is daily aware of his learning differences. If he is not given proper instruction, he will continue to experience failure with traditional curriculum; this is devastating emotionally. The label is the ticket to appropriate help. It is probably better than the internal label of "failure" that the student may assign to himself with no intervention.

THE TEAM MEETING

At the team meeting, everyone who is interested in helping the student gathers. This includes parents and anyone the parents wish to invite, such as an advocate or legal representative, and school personnel who either are involved with the student's program or participated in the evaluation. If the student is at least fourteen years old, he is also invited to attend. An administrator from the school must be in attendance, as well as a person who can provide information on special education services.

The testing results are explained, and people are asked to contribute any information that may be helpful in determining eligibility for services. If it is decided by the team that the student qualifies for services, and the parents agree that they want their child to receive these services, the team then discusses the best way to provide this help. Usually, the team decides on the amount of time required for special services, the type of service required, and where these services will be provided. Staff positions are usually named as service providers instead of individual people; for example, it can be stated that the occupational therapist will work with the student twice a week for half-hour sessions each time. In some schools, the Individual Educational Plan (IEP) is written at the team meeting. Usually, however, the special education teacher and other service providers write their sections of this document later and then confer with parents regarding the specifics of the plan.

The most important aspect of the team meeting is the word "team." Everyone at this meeting knows the student from a slightly different perspective. Every person, therefore, can contribute something unique as eligibility and appropriate services are being discussed. Team meetings should be democratic meetings: Every person has the same opportunity and responsibility to freely discuss the student's needs and to make sure that he receives the best possible care.

THE INDIVIDUAL EDUCATIONAL PLAN (IEP)

Teachers and parents alike are often intimidated by the IEP because it looks very formal and is, in fact, a legal document. The specific formats of IEPs vary from place to place, but they all contain the following elements:

- where the service will be provided
- what type of professional will provide the service
- how much service will be provided
- information on the current functioning level of the student, including any relevant test data
- information on the learning strengths and weaknesses of the student, which often includes information on social and emotional needs
- goals for the student
- objectives, that delineate how the goals will be reached
- any special educational programs or methodology that will be used
- when particular goals and objectives are to be met
- any modifications that need to be made; for example, modifications in standardized testing, transportation, or physical education requirements

The goals and objectives are the heart of the IEP. This is where the areas of need are defined and the teaching methodology to help meet these needs is outlined. Students can have any number of goals. Some examples are:

1. Michael will develop his reading skills.
2. Michael will develop his handwriting skills.
3. Michael will improve his study skills.
4. Michael will improve his writing skills.

Objectives tell how to meet these needs. For example, some objectives that could be written for Michael's goal 4 might be:

1. Michael will be able to write sentences on a wide variety of topics.
2. Michael will be able to write a structured paragraph consisting of a topic sentence, three supporting detail sentences, and an ending sentence.
3. Michael will be able to self-edit his writing for beginning capitalization and ending punctuation marks.
4. Michael will be able to recognize nouns and verbs.
5. Michael will learn keyboarding skills, including writing the alphabet, words, and simple sentences.

The goals and objectives do not have to be complicated. They should be simple and clear and provide a type of map that documents what will be worked on and how this will be done. The details should just support, not overrun, the more important general statements about learning style and methodology.

WORK BEGINS: HOW TO KNOW IF INTERVENTION IS WORKING

Once the parents have signed the IEP, the student can begin to receive services. For students with dyslexia, this is an important step, but it is only the beginning. Because the needs of students with dyslexia are so diverse, educational programs need to be carefully planned. The IEP outlines the basic areas of work and methodology, but diagnostic teaching must be undertaken for every individual as the work progresses: The teacher needs to carefully watch pacing, which multimodality techniques work best, the need for review and practice, and other factors. In the methodology chapters of this resource, more specific information on diagnostic teaching for each academic area will be provided.

Observable progress takes time, but generally, there should be some marked improvement in basic skills in six months. The biggest indicator of whether the intervention is working is the student himself. Is he feeling more positive about himself and his work? Is he willingly participating in his special work? Some older students who have experienced a lot of failure may repress even this indicator. They may be feeling so badly about themselves from the past that it is difficult for them to see real progress now. These students have to fight against the feeling that they will never "get it." It will take more time, but eventually, they will be able to see their own progress.

How long should intervention continue? Every student is different, but as a general rule, most students with mild dyslexia require at least two years of special teaching. Students with moderate to severe dyslexia sometimes need special education services throughout their school careers.

What, in the end, can be expected of a student who has received good intervention? Generally, most professionals agree on the following:

- Students with dyslexia can learn to read.
- They can become good mathematicians.
- They can learn to spell, even though they do not usually become great spellers. With the advent of computer spell checks, however, this is less of a burden.
- They can be successful in most academic areas, but may have a weakness in foreign languages.
- They can be successful in college.
- They can be successful in adult life.

THE ANNUAL REVIEW AND THE THREE-YEAR REEVALUATION

THE ANNUAL REVIEW

After the student has been receiving services for a year, the team reconvenes to discuss the program. This is a time to reassess the level, type, and setting of services. The annual review is just as important as the initial team meeting. If the student's program has been going well, especially, people are more relaxed at the annual review and the tendency is just to continue the existing plan. Things may have changed, however. Because the student is beginning to read and write, for example, he may now be able to focus on other areas such as keyboarding and organizational skills. It may be time to work specifically on independent study skills.

Once again, the annual review is a place for people who care about the student's welfare to gather and to be honest with one another about the student's program. Often, the more information that is shared, the better the educational plan becomes.

THE THREE-YEAR REEVALUATION

Every three years, students who are receiving special education services are reevaluated. Many of the tests that were administered at the time of diagnosis will be given again. This is a good opportunity to assess progress and current needs. Even though it is time consuming for the school system and for the student, this three-year reevaluation provides a good opportunity to stand back and really look at what has happened academically for the student.

INDEPENDENT EVALUATIONS

Parents have the right to have a child evaluated by a professional who is not employed by the school system if they feel that the evaluation done by the school is incomplete. School systems often pay for this evaluation, but sometimes parents pay for it themselves. They often do this because they are then able to freely choose the professional who will do the evaluation, and they are not obliged to share the results with the school.

DUE PROCESS

The federal law IDEA stipulates that parents have the right to a due process hearing if they feel that the child's rights under the law have not been met. The law outlines general principles for this hearing, but states define the specific regulations. Parents have to request such a hearing in writing, and school systems are obliged to process these requests in a timely way.

Often, states offer an opportunity for mediation prior to due process hearings. A mediation officer presides, while teachers, parents, and other relevant professionals discuss the history of the student's academic experience. Mediation, in many cases, can resolve the issues.

TIPS FOR TEACHERS AND PARENTS

- It is empowering to know the specific regulations that govern special education services. Teachers then clearly know their responsibilities, and parents become aware of their rights and the rights of their children. Contact the principal of your school or the special education director and ask for the local regulations. Then, contact your state department of education to get a copy of the state regulations.

- When you are carrying out initial observations of a student, look for his strengths as well as for his weak areas. These strengths can provide clues to successful methodology.

- Prior to referral, during a time when the student's privacy is being protected, ask him about some of the factors you have observed. For example, you could say, "I noticed that you didn't really want to start on that math work this afternoon. Did it feel too hard? Or were you just tired?" This conversation needs to be very sensitively done, and you should not talk with your student in this way if you sense that he will perceive it as criticism. If the student is comfortable speaking with you, however, valuable information can be obtained.

- It's true that the squeaky wheel gets the grease, and all too often in schools, the student with the behavior problem gets noticed first for services. This is especially documented for girls with dyslexia, who can go unnoticed for long periods of time because they are well behaved and quiet. The student with dyslexia has significant needs that should be addressed, whether they are causing problems in the classroom or not. You must advocate strongly for them.

- School psychologists, special education teachers, and other professionals can be overworked and therefore unable to serve students in a timely way. If this is your situation, do not put off referring a student because of a backlog of cases. Documentation that there may be a need for more personnel is important, and school psychologists and others will be glad of the extra help it may produce. Your primary responsibility is to advocate for the student.

INTERVIEW WITH FRAN

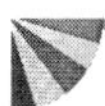

Here, Fran, who is an advocate who spoke in Chapter 2, talks about the law and other aspects of special education.

What are some of the best things that you think have happened since the IDEA was created?

Well, it gives both teachers and parents an avenue for training, for appropriate identification, and it also has encouraged a lot more research. I don't think we would know today what we do if it weren't for the law.

What makes a team meeting effective?

It's effective if you're all on the same team—if you're really, truly looking to see what's not working and what pieces must be there to have the child benefit from his education. And there are certainly some schools that I go into where we're all on the same team; there aren't sides at the table.

I was at a team meeting in which we were discussing a child who has severe language needs. I had been involved with the family for a long time, and things were working. Things were working for him. We were getting trained people to do things.

Then he was in an automobile accident, and he had a head injury. It magnified everything that was wrong before. And we were still working, but with all kinds of puzzles. The program was falling apart, and we couldn't figure it out. The kid kept falling asleep in school.

We had a new player on the team who said, "He's just not trying," but there were a lot of people sitting at this table. As we sat around we kept saying, "Why is it breaking down? Why is he falling asleep?"

I said, "There's got to be a pattern here. When did it start breaking down?" We went back and analyzed it. There had been a second automobile accident that had caused anxiety and frustration, so they had upped the boy's medication level. It ended up that that was exactly when things fell apart. And then, suddenly, things fell into place. Nobody was to blame.

Everyone on the team was saying, "Where did you see it break down? When did this happen?" By pulling, pulling, pulling . . . that's how the team should work. It should be a puzzle. And you're not blaming anyone. It's not an indictment of the teacher or the kid. It's a puzzle. This is where it's breaking down, and this is what he needs.

It was the medication that was causing the problem?

Yes. Then we were able to change his schedule and to work around the medication issue, and now we have a plan. We may still have some glitches, but now we work as a team. It's an effective team, because everybody has some piece to share. Before, until we got all the pieces on the table, we couldn't find the answer.

What do you think are the critical aspects of an effective IEP?

The law is wonderful, it's absolutely fantastic, and if you go back and study the history of it and its development, it's wonderful. You've got to wipe the slate clean, and you start from what the needs are. What are the identified strengths and weaknesses, and then how are you going to address them? And don't worry about, well, we have block scheduling or we can't do this. You first have to identify what's not working, how are we going to fix it, and last, get to placement.

How do you know when an intervention is working?

Oh, it's easy. Kids know. I have a client who is in a public high school, who was reading in the first or second percentile. Bright girl. She had gone to this tutor for a couple of months, and her mother said, "We're going to take the summer off." The girl said, "No, you're not taking Juanita away from me."

I find that parents will say, "I don't want to put them through more testing." I've never had the kids—any of the people I've worked with—have a problem with an incredible amount of testing if they feel that it's coming up with an answer and they're going to learn to read. Kids know when they're going to learn to read. They can tell you if you know what you're doing.

You can take them right back to the beginning. Usually, schools don't go back far enough. They say, "Well, you're in fifth grade, so you'd better do fifth grade curriculum." Instead, they should say, "You don't know the alphabet. We have to go back and teach the alphabet. And kids will go back.

I've seen kids in college who literally cannot write the alphabet or repeat the alphabet. Or they have to do the alphabet song in order to do the alphabet. You can go back and teach them the pieces that are missing, because one of the characteristics is that we (people with dyslexia) have strengths and weaknesses, and we have knowledge, and we're all above average in intelligence, so we may have pieces that are intact and pieces that aren't. You can go back to the very beginning, and you must. If you don't go back to phonemic awareness, if that's where it's breaking down, it's like building a house starting with the roof and working down. The whole thing falls down. That's what happens with reading. If you don't start at the beginning and fill in the holes, the house won't stand.

CHAPTER 4

INTERVENTION

HOW MUCH INTERVENTION IS NEEDED?

Most students with dyslexia require some form of intervention. Some of them are so bright and have such a mild form of dyslexia that they can cope with traditional curriculum. This does not mean, however, that they can flourish. As teachers, we need to look carefully at each of our students and advocate for the level of intervention that will not just help them use compensatory strategies but will allow them to function at their true intellectual potential.

As a general rule, many students with mild to moderate dyslexia can show real progress with two to three hours a week of direct instruction by a person knowledgeable about the learning style. Of course, there is no magic about this number, but it is a good place to start. As we look at a student to decide specifically how much intervention is needed, we need to consider:

- the degree to which the student has the learning style
- how many academic areas are affected by the learning style
- the emotional and behavioral issues affecting the student

A high degree of all of the above requires greater amounts of intervention. One more thing needs to be considered, too: the age of the student. Usually, because of developmental level and attention span, younger children tend to profit from shorter, more frequent intervention sessions.

WHERE CAN INSTRUCTION BE PROVIDED?

THE REGULAR CLASSROOM—THE INCLUSION MODEL

Students with dyslexia usually have at least normal intellectual potential, and it therefore makes sense to keep them, as much as is possible, in the regular classroom. The inclusion model has been a popular model in public education for the past few years.

The advantages to students are that they can be educated with their peers and that they are not singled out by the larger community as different.

In the inclusion model, the classroom teacher is usually supported by a special education teacher. This person helps the classroom teacher plan appropriate curriculum modifications, and/or works with the student directly. The special education teacher can support what is happening in the classroom, and provide specialized instruction for the learning style.

Having a student with dyslexia in the regular classroom requires a great deal of time, commitment, and work. For the student with this learning style, it is critically important to keep the following in mind as instruction is provided:

> ***Good classrooms are often happy, bustling places.*** Since many students with dyslexia have auditory issues, they need to work in quiet environments, especially on things which are often difficult for them such as phonemic awareness.
>
> ***Good classrooms often have exciting and stimulating visual environments.*** Since many students with dyslexia are easily distractible, it is important to provide a relatively stimulus free setting when they are receiving specialized instruction in their areas of difficulty,
>
> ***Students with dyslexia sometimes require instruction that looks developmentally immature.*** For example, because of phonemic awareness issues, they often require multisensory work with phonics. Sometimes, blocks that represent sounds are used. This can be embarrassing for the older student when her peers are watching her work, and, therefore, care must be taken that her privacy is assured during this work time.

Individual Tutorial Work Outside the Regular Classroom

Here, the student stays with her peers during most of the school day but has regular scheduled sessions with a special education teacher outside of classroom. A private, quiet space and sensitivity to avoiding disruption of the schedule needs to be provided. This can be an extremely effective model, especially if all the teachers involved with the student discuss her program and needs, and if classroom modifications are made.

Instruction in the Resource Room

Here, the student spends a part of her day in a separate classroom. The advantage of this model is that, if the dyslexic learning style is affecting several academic areas, the student can receive appropriate instruction in the many different areas. If there are other students who require the same type and amount of intervention in the resource room, they can be placed in small groups, and this model can be highly effective.

Instruction in the Self-contained Classroom

This can be an effective model for those students who have a high degree of dyslexia, and who have most academic areas affected. Programs can be carefully planned to group students for instruction and, also, to provide some individual intervention. The total program, including art, science, and physical education, can be planned around general principles that meet the specific needs of students with dyslexia. The disadvantage of this model is that students are singled out as having special needs by the larger school community. It is important in this case to plan carefully for the student's transition back into regular programs.

Instruction in a Special School

Some public and private schools specialize in working with students with dyslexia. These schools can be helpful for students who have significant degrees of dyslexia that significantly affect their total school experience. Some students require not only individual work in reading but also individual or very small group work in spelling, writing, and math. All the academic areas need to be carefully structured and presented in multisensory ways. For these students, specialized schools can be very effective. The disadvantage is that students have to leave their former school community, and again, the transition back needs to be carefully planned.

WHAT SPECIALISTS CAN HELP?

This resource gives basic information on providing appropriate instruction for students with dyslexia. Some clinicians, however, have specialized in the field and can provide important additional services. They not only work with students but can also consult with teachers to make sure that the total intervention plan is optimally effective.

Tutors and Educational Therapists

If the existing IEP plan does not seem to be working, it can be very helpful to enlist the help of a specialized tutor or educational therapist. These highly experienced and credentialed people have worked for years with students with this unique learning style. They are able, therefore, not only to provide highly skilled instruction but also to work with an individual student in a diagnostic teaching way and to provide good information about the best methodology for teachers to use in other settings. Communication and coordination are key.

Some tutors have received specialized training in programs such as the Lindamood Phoneme Sequencing Program, discussed in more depth on pages 70 and 71 of this resource. If a student has severe difficulty with auditory discrimination, such a tutor can provide very valuable help.

DEVELOPMENTAL OPTOMETRISTS

There has been controversy for many years regarding these specially trained optometrists. Many people have thought that dyslexia was only a language based issue, and that optometrists who claimed to help by offering vision training were optimistic but unrealistic. Recent research at Stanford University, however—even though it was done on a small sample—indicates that vision may play a part for some students.

Developmental optometrists claim that special vision training helps the eye muscles work more efficiently and effectively. They state that this work can help students' eyes work together better, focus more easily, and move from left to right more efficiently. As further research is conducted, more information will surely be gained about the effectiveness of vision training.

SPEECH AND LANGUAGE CLINICIANS

Students with significant speech and language issues usually need intervention from a speech and language therapist. These professionals are highly trained and usually qualify for state accreditation. Students can need help in one or all of the following areas:

- Articulation, or the ability to pronounce words correctly.
- Receptive language, or the ability to absorb language. Listening skills can be affected.
- Expressive language, or the ability to speak fluently and naturally. The ability to speak in grammatically correct English can be affected, as well as the ability to think of and say a specific known word.

Speech and language clinicians not only provide direct intervention but can also give good recommendations for instructional adaptations.

OCCUPATIONAL THERAPISTS

Some students with dyslexia have significant difficulty with fine motor skills. This can sometimes be remediated with good instruction, as when a fine, multisensory handwriting program is used to teach cursive writing. The severity of the need of some students in this area, however, requires additional work. They can also have difficulty not only with fine-motor tasks but with gross-motor tasks and balance, as well. Motor coordination of the big muscle groups can be problematic, and this makes sports and other supposedly "fun" activities very difficult.

Some students are highly sensitive to touch; they dislike being physically touched at all—even in socially acceptable ways—and they can dislike touching things like clay in art class.

Occupational therapists are highly trained and provide specific types of exercises and instruction to help with these problems. As with other professionals, they can also make recommendations for classroom modifications.

OTHER ISSUES REGARDING SCHOOL PLACEMENT

SCHOOL ENTRY

Students with dyslexia are sometimes developmentally younger than their same-age peers. For this reason, it can be a good idea for a child who is suspected of having dyslexia and who appears to be immature to stay in a nursery school program for an extra year before entering kindergarten. Doctors, school psychologists, and special education teachers can be consulted about this decision, and screening for kindergarten readiness can be carried out. If issues such as speech and language problems are shown on the screening, appropriate services should be initiated prior to the child's formally entering school.

RETENTION

"Staying back" is not a good option for students with dyslexia. They will not progress with another year of traditional curriculum; rather, they will progress only with appropriate intervention. Once this is provided, they can make excellent progress and, therefore, the need for retention is gone.

The one place where retention can be considered is in kindergarten because of developmental issues. One possibility, for example, is to "promote" a child from a half-day kindergarten program to a full-day kindergarten program, along with making modifications to fit the child's learning style. A great deal of attention should be placed on how the child and the child's family, including her siblings, feel about her not moving directly on to first grade.

INTERVIEW WITH FRAN

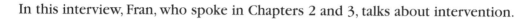

In this interview, Fran, who spoke in Chapters 2 and 3, talks about intervention.

Do you think it matters where the intervention is provided, assuming that the teacher is using good teaching methods?

It doesn't matter if it's good intervention and it's working.

What about the time of day?

It depends on the students, but if you're doing it after school, and they're exhausted from trying to hold it together in school, they're not going to get as much value as they would if they had had it first thing in the morning. Now, some kids are tired in the morning and take longer to wake up because of ADD or something like that. You have to time it. If you're going to put the time and resources and money into it, you should do it at the optimum period of the day so that you can get the best results, and then you can do it for the shortest amount of time. It should be really intensive, because the whole purpose of special education is to get these kids out, not to have it go on for 12 years. If you look at the schools that are successful, it's the level of intensity that makes the difference.

When do you think intervention should begin?

Probably at six months. (Fran laughs here). All the research shows that it should be very early.

What do you believe are some of the advantages of early intervention?

You prevent children from having negative self-image esteem issues. It's also much cheaper.

You should also train regular teachers. You could have early intervention in preschool or kindergarten, and in my opinion, you should be able to have most kids out by the time they reach first or second grade. You would eliminate 95 percent of your population. Some kids are so severe that they are going to require intervention for a longer period of time, but that's a tiny percentage.

Who are some of the specialists that you find helpful?

You need speech pathologists, occupational therapists who know about sensory integration, and psychologists.

Language is incredibly important, and you need a speech pathologist who is trained in language, not articulation. It's important to have a speech pathologist, because there's a natural continuum of language. It starts with oral language, both receptive and expressive; then it moves to reading and then to written expression.

If it is breaking down for students in oral language, if you start with reading and don't fix the oral language, it's going to be much more difficult for them to learn and to comprehend and to make proper interpretations of language. They don't understand certain aspects. Their vocabulary is going to be small. You must fix the oral language, so you need a speech pathologist.

You often need a psychologist or a social worker or some kind of therapist who can help students to understand their disorder; to understand how to explain it, both to themselves and to others; and to figure out ways to handle stress. There may be family issues; there may be peer issues. Often these kids have problems reading social language, body language, so there are all kinds of issues like that.

Some of these kids are wonderful athletes; others are not. They may have gross- or fine-motor problems, so they may need more physical education.

Another thing that I find is that a kid may have problems with labels in his shirts. That's one of the questions I always ask parents. You'll find that many students with dyslexia also have all kinds of issues with sensory integration. They don't like to wear sweaters, or their socks are too tight.

Are you talking about tactile defensiveness?

Yes. That's the kid who's always getting in trouble because he's pushing the kid next to him in line. In kindergarten, the teacher's always pulling him out of line. Put him at the head of the line or at the end of the line, or have him be an assistant, but see that he's not too close.

Other people are experiencing it as aggression, and he's experiencing it as being touched. He doesn't like to be touched.

Exactly. And if you see a child who puts his head down when he's writing, he's not getting the information from his fingertips, which constitutes the fastest way to the brain. He is using his eyes to draw. Instead of writing, he's actually drawing the letters, using his eyes to dictate where the pencil goes. There are all kinds of signs. Then you need an occupational therapist who is trained in sensory integration.

What do you think about keeping children home an extra year before kindergarten, if they have difficulties?

What you want is early intervention, so you want them in school as soon as possible. You want as much stimulation, as much development of vocabulary as you can give them. It's not going to go away. They're not going to outgrow it. If you say that they're too young for school, you're actually losing out on time.

The only way that keeping them out would make sense is if you had somebody tutoring them. Sometimes the kids appear immature, and we think—and sometimes we're told—that they'll outgrow it, but they won't. So another year isn't the answer. Getting a proper program in place is the answer. Once they've started school, holding them back is a disaster.

Is there ever a reason to retain a student?

No. Interestingly, the School Psychologists Association has a very strong statement that says it is reprehensible to hold a kid back. If, let's say, he was in an automobile accident or he was hospitalized for six months, that would be a reason to hold him back, because he actually missed school.

If a child is struggling that badly, you must radically increase services. What you're doing is not working. It may mean a different school, a different placement, or highly individualized treatment or remediation.

Would you talk about teachers whom you admire, who you feel have been very effective working with students with dyslexia?

They keep looking. They teach in a diagnostic way, and it never even enters their heads that a student isn't motivated, isn't trying, isn't able. If certain programs they use aren't working, they go out and find other programs that they think will be more effective. Effective teachers constantly ask, "How can I get through?" They believe that there's an answer, and they keep on.

CHAPTER 5

TEN GENERAL PRINCIPLES OF INSTRUCTION

When we think of teaching students with dyslexia, we have to distinguish between accommodation and remediation. The former is the process of making modifications to traditional curriculum. The latter is the process of providing direct, specific instruction in the area of weakness. Most students with dyslexia require both types of instruction, especially if they are in classroom settings for much of their school day.

This chapter offers general principles that are essential for good remediation. These same principles, however, also apply to well-thought-out accommodation plans.

1. INVOLVE THE STUDENT

The first and most basic principle is to discuss all aspects of the educational plan with the student. All students, even those with typical learning styles profit from this, but the student with dyslexia really needs to be involved with the process of his own instruction.

Think of a general characteristic of the dyslexic learning style: People are global learners, and therefore learn best when small pieces of information are placed in a larger context. They tend to focus best when interested and when actively engaged. For these reasons, it is important to discuss the following:

- ***The Goals for the Instruction.*** Tell your student what you hope to accomplish, and ask him what he wants. If he has trouble telling you this at first, tell him that it is sometimes difficult to establish goals, but that you will be periodically checking in with him about them, because what he wishes to accomplish with this instruction is very important to you. Sometimes, it is difficult for students to express goals if they do not know and trust you yet, or if they don't feel hopeful about their progress. It is a big risk to state openly what they want from the instruction. If handled sensitively over a period of time, however, this process of establishing goals can be extremely helpful.

- ***The Teaching Methods.*** Quickly tell your student how you will be approaching your job of teaching, and give him the rationale. For example, for spelling you could say, "We are going to study the structure of the English language, so that you'll know the logic of how it's constructed. That way, you won't have to rely on your memory for individual words all the time." This explanation should be a short overview of the general approach.
- ***The Student's Progress.*** Ask your student how he feels he is doing. Which parts of the lesson are difficult for him, and which are easiest? Does he have a sense of what particular activities seem to help him learn best? Your student can provide a wealth of good information concerning the particulars of his learning program. If he is feeling discouraged about his own progress, it very important for you to know this and to allow him time to speak about these feelings. You may also need to adapt your teaching methods.

2. USE MULTISENSORY TEACHING METHODS

Much traditional instruction is based on the linguistic modality. The student sits passively while the teacher gives him information. Discussion often occurs. Then, he reads about the topic and, ultimately, either writes a report or passes a written test. Students with dyslexia need a much more active and interactive road to learning. It is helpful for them to feel objects, to see and hear material, to write down what they are learning, and, sometimes, to write about it. They can use their kinesthetic sense, as when they are pantomiming a vocabulary word. Occasionally, where appropriate, the sense of taste is even utilized.

The Orton-Gillingham approach to reading and spelling was a pioneer in championing the use of multisensory methods for teaching. With this method, students see, hear, say, and write what they are learning. As much reinforcement as possible is provided.

The particulars of how to utilize multisensory techniques for teaching specific academic areas is provided in the next few chapters. In general, however, whenever you are providing instruction, ask yourself the following question: "Am I talking a lot while my student sits and listens?" If the answer is yes, you need to redesign the program.

3. TEACH STUDENTS TO USE LOGIC RATHER THAN ROTE MEMORY

A common area of weakness for students with dyslexia is short-term and long-term memory, especially of things that do not have much meaning. A common area of strength is good intelligence. For this reason, cognition is used wherever possible to teach students the systems of things; for example, as in spelling, in which the structure of the English language is taught. Students learn about the six syllable types, and about spelling rules that allow them to figure out correct spelling, as opposed to relying only on their memories. Because approximately 85 percent of the English language is phonetically regular, they can rely on their knowledge of the language for most words. They can then use either their memory or compensatory strategies such as dictionaries and computer spell checks for the remaining 15 percent. To summarize, they learn patterns, rather than having to memorize hundreds of isolated words.

People with dyslexia tend to think in patterns and generalities. This strength of their learning style, therefore, can greatly help them deal with a number of details, with which they are often less comfortable.

4. PRESENT MATERIAL SEQUENTIALLY

Start from the very beginning and build slowly. A common metaphor that often helps students—especially older ones—is to tell them that you are building a house of knowledge together. Whenever a house is built, it is critically important that the foundation be strong and solid. You are therefore going to make sure that there are no holes in their foundations of knowledge. Once they have a solid foundation, they will be able to learn with much less effort. While talking about this, it can even be helpful to draw a little house to emphasize your point.

The house-building metaphor, or one like it, is actually quite important to present. It helps students understand why you are starting at the basics. Some teachers of traditional curriculum feel that students need to be challenged, and that they are not learning unless they are working extremely hard and feeling slightly overwhelmed. Your students—especially older ones—may have been exposed to this philosophy. Even though they have suffered with it, they also may have accepted the basic tenet- that learning occurs most readily when the work feels hard. Thus, they need the more accurate information that people usually learn best and fastest when material is presented in sequential steps. One step builds on another in a cumulative way.

5. PRESENT MATERIAL IN SMALL UNITS

Once again, we are opposing a common cultural point of view that "more is better." For the student with dyslexia, less is definitely better. If a lot of material is presented at one time, his usual response is either to act out or to tune out. He will probably remember none of the material.

It is far better to present a small amount of material and to make sure that he is completely comfortable with it, and then to move on to the next small piece of material. If you are moving too slowly and presenting too little for a student, and he really can absorb material at a faster rate, he will let you know, and you can then alter your lesson planning. The most important thing is for you to keep open communication with your student about how quickly you both are working, and to check with him regularly about his comfort level with the pacing of the work.

6. PRACTICE, PRACTICE, PRACTICE, AND REVIEW

It is essential to provide many opportunities for reinforcement of material presented. In his remedial work, especially, a student is working in an area that is difficult for him. He therefore needs many different types of chances to review and practice what he has learned.

Often, a good lesson begins with a review of what was presented in prior lessons. A student is sometimes asked to discuss with the teacher something he has learned. If he has already talked about it and written about it, perhaps it's now time to draw a picture or present a short drama about the topic. It is especially good to provide a wide variety of types of experiences, utilizing many different modalities, that will reinforce what he is learning.

7. HELP STUDENTS ORGANIZE TIME AND SPACE

Many students with dyslexia have difficulty with organization of both time and space. Helping them with this issue not only avoids problems but also gives them that important overview of the work that puts details in their proper places. It is good to provide assistance with organization in the following areas:

- ***The Daily Lesson.*** It is surprisingly helpful to tell students what you will be working on during that session. For example, if it's a writing class that will last an hour, you can say, "First, we'll write a list, then we'll work on our paragraphs, and then, Sam, would you like to work on your report on bears? Great. I'll read to you for about ten minutes at the end of class." This simple telling of what will happen provides a predictable and safe environment for learning.
- ***The Work Space.*** The classroom needs to be orderly, with extraneous objects or papers placed neatly in appropriate categories. This not only models spending time on organization but it also helps cut down on distracting stimuli.
- ***Students' Daily Work.*** It is recommended that students keep their work in a three-ring binder, which is divided by tabs into appropriate sections. Every time they finish a paper, they can place it in the right place in their notebooks, noting the type of work they have just finished and the date of the work. This models spending time on organization on a regular basis. It also gives students practice on how to categorize and organize details into a larger whole. Ideally, a separate three-ring notebook should be kept for every subject area.
- ***Long-term and Complex Work Assignments.*** The best thing to do is to simply discuss the total project and to make a plan of the steps that need to be

accomplished in order to complete the project. Tell your student that, once he has started work, he can change the particulars of this plan. Tell him that beginning a long project is hard, and it makes it a lot easier to spend some time in this kind of preparation. If the student is capable of writing down this plan in sequential steps, ask him to do so. If not, you should write it out and give it to him to keep in his notebook. Then, especially as he begins work, refer often to the plan. This technique not only helps your student be successful with the particular project but it also teaches him how to approach a difficult assignment in future times when he will have to do so independently.

- ***Multiple Asignments.*** For remediation work, you occasionally may assign more than one task for older and advanced students, for example, for homework. The purpose of this is mostly to teach them how to handle more than one task. With accommodation work, however, especially with older students, multiple assignments will be a major thing you will have to deal with. Unfortunately, many students with dyslexia have a tendency to forget or lose things, especially objects of potentially low value such as homework notebooks. For this reason, the traditional methods often don't work. There is no magic in this area. It is simply important to keep trying systems until something works. Will a special notebook with a beautiful cover be more loss resistant, for example? Do you need to watch the student actually place the homework notebook in his backpack? Does it help for him to check with a buddy at the end of the day to make sure he is bringing home all necessary books and papers? In time, something will work.

8. INDIVIDUALIZE INSTRUCTION

Students with dyslexia are so different that they cannot be placed into convenient slots for educational programming. In fact, most good approaches recognize this by presenting methods, as opposed to rigid programs. Students need to work at their own pace, utilizing their strong modalities to remediate their weaknesses. Even if you have a group of only two students at a similar level, you may have to make some alterations in programming for each student. Lesson planning has to be individualized for each subject area taught, also, because a student's needs in one area may be different from those in another. Keep evaluating the lesson plan, so that it continues to be optimally effective.

9. ALWAYS BE AWARE OF THE EMOTIONAL CLIMATE

Most students with dyslexia started out experiencing failure with academics and, consequently, have great insecurities about their ability to succeed. Students with dyslexia also work very hard, especially in a well-designed remediation program.

Occasionally, it is difficult for them to maintain this hopeful effort; their hard work seems to be bearing fruit, but it seems to be taking so long. They are also inclined to judge their performance against that of same-age peers in the classroom.

These negative feelings are very painful and very real. As you work with a student, be aware of his emotional tone. Is he suddenly starting to be late for his work session? Is he withdrawn and anxious? Is he starting to wander around the room, playing with objects? Is he expressing anger toward fellow students? All of these are signs that something may be amiss.

You can say to your student something like this: "I've been noticing that you've been late a lot lately. I think that maybe you're tired of doing this work. Do you want to talk about it?" In Chapter 16 of this resource, emotional issues and how to deal with them are discussed in more detail. Put simply, however, it often helps to recognize the student's unusual behavior, and to say what you think it may indicate. Then, ask if the student wishes to discuss the subject further. Be careful not to tell the student why he is acting the way he is. (You could be wrong. He could be experiencing difficulty at home; for example, a parents' divorce that is still a secret outside the family.) Also, respect his privacy if he does not wish to discuss his feelings. Your attempt to reach out to him in a nurturing and understanding way will tell him that you care about him, and this can help build a positive relationship.

10. LAUGH A LOT

This may seem to be a frivolous general principle, but it is actually very important. It is hard work to remediate language and other difficulties—both for the student and for the teacher. Most of the time is spent in highly focused, highly structured study, and it has to be this way in order to be effective.

People tend to learn best when they are relaxed and comfortable. Humor can be very helpful in breaking the fatigue and tension of a long, hard-working session. When teacher and students are laughing together, everybody relaxes. For this reason, make an effort occasionally to provide something funny. Look in newspapers, for example, for humorous stories about people or animals; or have a book like *Where the Sidewalk Ends: Poems and Drawings* by Shel Silverstein (Harper-Collins, 1974). This book can offer many humorous moments to be shared with your students.

All of these principles are simple and basic, but they are also very powerful. Use them, and your students will be successful.

TIPS FOR TEACHERS

- ***Provide Pencils.*** As students with dyslexia often have a tendency to lose things, it can become a major issue for them always to come to class with a sharpened pencil. Take away the issue, and focus on the instruction for the day.

When the time is right, you can work on organizational and "not losing things" skills as a separate and distinct goal.

- ***Read Aloud.*** You can read aloud in all subject areas, not just reading. A sophisticated picture book such as *The Red Comb* by Fernando Pico, and illustrated by Maria Antonia Ordonez (BridgeWater Books, 1995), which tells of slavery in Puerto Rico in the 1800s, can, for example, be an excellent stimulus for discussion in a social studies or history class. Perhaps students would like to discuss the probability of a certain event occurring in a given story (a math-related issue). Reading aloud offers reinforcement, a change of pace, relationship building, and excellent stimulation for new ideas.
- ***Take an Occasional Break and Be More Informal.*** Plant a bulb, or look at and read a group of interesting nonfiction pictorial books from a library. Students with dyslexia desperately need structure and consistency, but sometimes they also need a change. Providing such a positive diversion helps them resume work with renewed energy.
- ***Go to Tag Sales.*** Students with dyslexia need to use manipulative materials in most subject areas. If purchased in conventional ways, these materials can be very expensive. Tag and garage sales, therefore, are an excellent alternative where you can find all sorts of wonderful and interesting objects for very little money.
- ***Provide Legitimate Outlets for Extra Energy.*** Because many students with dyslexia are very active physically, it's important not to have that become an issue during lessons. Plan for some physical movement during the session. Can the student try to pantomime a word that is being studied, for example? Does the chalkboard need a quick, vigorous cleaning?
- ***Respond to Positive Efforts and Behaviors.*** Try to ignore inappropriate behavior as much as possible. Paying attention to, and even giving verbal praise to the positive behaviors helps to reinforce them.

INTERVIEW WITH DANIEL

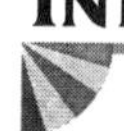

Daniel is a 15-year-old boy who enjoys playing basketball, making trails in the woods, and writing. He is currently a student at a small private school for students with special needs.

What advice would you give to a new teacher, who just graduated from college, on how to be a good teacher?

Don't be too strict. Be a nice teacher. Be very clear about what the assignment is, and what to do. Um, like . . . be clear about what you should do and have a good class. Do good things, like write a story or something for English class. You can tell about it and do a little project on it. That's a good way to start. And give good courage to them and tell them things.

How should they give good courage to their students ?

Tell them they're doing a good job, and tell them that they're good students and they're doing a good job. And teach them, teach them before you do it, like do it pretty slow and tell them one step at a time.

What if there's a kid who's having trouble? What would you tell that teacher to do?

I'd tell that teacher to just give a little bit more attention to him, if he has any questions, and let him, if he needs to, like, think it over. Let him leave class and go to study hall and try to think it over and try to do his work, if he has a hard time doing it in class.

Why would study hall help?

Because if you're by yourself, you can concentrate more. If it's reading and it's a noisy classroom, you can concentrate in the study hall because there won't be all that noise going on.

What if the kid was saying, "I can't do this. This is too hard for me." What would you tell the teacher to do?

I'd just go through it. I'd go through the steps, go through what to do and try to teach him how to do it.

What kind of projects are helpful?

Like doing stuff on trees and regular stuff. How a septic system works, and how things work out in the world. And for math, do word problems that really happen out in the world. And do things like, teach the easier, instead of the really complicated things to start with, start with the easier ways. If there are easier ways to do the math, start with that, and then build up. Because there are many ways of doing things.

CHAPTER 6

TEACHING READING

Reading is a critical life skill, and the inability to read has emotional and social as well as academic and vocational ramifications. Reading is a part of everyday life, even for a child. She needs to read street signs, prepared food packages, menus, and directions for playing games. When a child sees these necessary words as confusing masses of unknown symbols instead of as understandable labels, this sets her apart from other children. Her peers can read; why can't she? The child all too often decides that it is because she is stupid.

RECOGNIZING THE READER WITH DYSLEXIA

Often, a child has already experienced a lot of frustration by the time it is established that she has dyslexia. For this reason, resistance to reading, and, in some extreme cases, even a phobia about print, is evident with many of these beginning readers. Try to place a book in the hands of such a child, and she may either try to talk with you at great length or play with objects in the room or (better still) attempt to go somewhere else, often under the table. Anything is better than looking at that confusing and changing mass of symbols.

Why is print so confusing? If you check, you will often find that she has no clear sense of the sounds associated with letters. This is particularly difficult in the English language because letters can represent more than one sound; for example, the letter "c" represents both /k/ and /s/. Also, the same sound can be represented by more than one letter, as when /f/ is called forth by "f" or "ph."

Most people with dyslexia need help with phonemic awareness. This is also sometimes referred to as phonological awareness. Phonemes are the smallest units of sound in English, such as /t/ and /e/. People with dyslexia often have difficulty recognizing and remembering which sounds are associated with which letters, knowing how many sounds there are in a word, and knowing the order of the sounds in the word. Thus, recognizing the relationships between sounds can be a real problem, as when they need to blend or otherwise combine sounds into syllables and words. In addition, people with dyslexia can have trouble with auditory discrimination, in other words, hearing the small differences between sounds.

Students with dyslexia sometimes experience visual confusion and do not see the small differences between letters and/or words. Letters are not always stable and can change, as when "b" is perceived as "d." Reversals can also occur with words, as when "saw" becomes "was." Also, visual memory can be weak, so it's hard to remember what a written word represents. This is particularly confusing as it relates to sight words like "the" and "said," in which the sounds associated with these words are unique.

By the time you meet them, some students with dyslexia may be reading a little; they may have relatively good visual skills, which gives them a limited sight vocabulary—a few words that they can consistently name in different contexts. This can be particularly confusing for a teacher, because these students *are* reading, but they don't seem to progress. Their reading is slow and labored, with many inaccurate guesses, especially on words that have little inherent meaning. Names of people or places that occur in text are completely beyond them.

These students are using their good intelligence and their relative strengths to compensate for their discomfort and difficulty with print. They are constantly searching for meaning clues, but only sometimes finding them. They are working unbelievably hard, looking for anything that will help them figure out what all those symbols mean. Is it any wonder that these students do not choose to read?

A few students with dyslexia progress to the point where they can read many individual words. Combining them, however, is difficult. These students concentrate so hard on decoding the words that they can't relax and think about what the sentences and paragraphs mean. Still others have eye-tracking problems; their eyes do not move comfortably and naturally from left to right, and from the end of one line of text down to the beginning of the next. This slows them down, because they have to concentrate on just staying properly placed on the page. In both of the abovementioned cases, reading comprehension suffers dramatically. To be able to understand what you've read, you have to be able to forget about the "job" of reading and concentrate instead on the concepts and information being presented.

THE METHODS OF TEACHING READING

There has been much controversy over the last few years regarding the most effective teaching method. One group believes that phonics should be the basis of any reading program. Thus, students should use the decoding of individual words as their primary cueing system for figuring out an unfamiliar word. The other group—often referred to as whole-language proponents—believes that meaning is the critical factor that should be focused upon. Students should think about what they are reading and make intelligent guesses about what an unfamiliar word might be. Whole-language proponents, therefore, state that students should use meaning cues as their primary cueing system. As a secondary cueing system, they should be aware of the syntax—in other words, the grammatical structure of English—in order to make good guesses about words.

A HISTORICAL PERSPECTIVE ON READING INSTRUCTION

Before we begin the discussion of the specifics of the teaching method that is recommended, it is helpful to look at what has come before. Many professional tutors and educational therapists who work with students with dyslexia have been highly influenced by the work of Dr. Samuel T. Orton, a neurologist. As early as 1919, he became interested in bright children who had trouble reading, and he began to study them. He teamed up with Anna Gillingham, a psychologist and Research Associate, and together, they developed a pioneering approach for teaching language skills (the Orton-Gillingham approach). One of their main contributions was to integrate the teaching of spelling, handwriting, and reading. Another hallmark of this approach is structured and sequential multisensory instruction. The phonemic code of the English language, or the ways that sounds and letters interact, is explicitly and carefully taught. There are many opportunities for drill and practice, and instruction is usually provided in a one-on-one setting. Students are taught to look at the phonetic structure of individual words as their primary cueing system.

In 1960, Anna Gillingham and Bessie Stillman created an instruction manual with educational materials for tutors. This important work has inspired many teachers, some of whom have adapted the approach for their own use. Others have been inspired to create their own programs based on this multisensory method.

Some well-known remedial programs that use the Orton-Gillingham approach as their model are Alphabetic Phonics, Recipe for Reading, the Slingerland Program, and the Wilson Reading System. These programs and others are discussed in more detail in *Dyslexia: Theory and Practice of Remedial Instruction*, 2d. ed., by Diana Brewster Clark and Joanna Kellogg Uhry (York Press, 1995).

WHICH READING METHOD WORKS BEST FOR STUDENTS WITH DYSLEXIA?

Most clinicians who teach students with dyslexia agree that there has to be explicit phonetic instruction for a program to be effective. This is supported by current research, which is identifying a lack of phonemic awareness as a critical issue in dyslexia. On the other hand, many clinicians are aware that an overreliance on the details of phonetic instruction to the exclusion of thinking about what the words and sentences mean can also create slow, stilted, unmotivated readers. Whole language philosophy has reminded us that reading involves all of the intellectual processes, and that the student has to think and care about what she is reading if she is going to be truly successful.

My belief is that all three cueing systems, the phonetic, the meaning, and the syntactic, should be taught simultaneously. In this way, students will learn to integrate them and use all three in a comfortable manner. But how do we integrate all three cueing systems so that we are teaching students to notice and rely on the phonetic structure of words while still thinking about the meaning and grammatical structure of what they are reading? It can be done. Always remember that dyslexia is a learning style with some significant weaknesses that require specific interventions. But there are also many important strengths associated with this learning style. Students are intelligent, and they have good common sense and logical thinking skills. They are able to see and relate to patterns. And they try very hard.

In the following pages, we will discuss the important aspects of instruction. We will begin with the all-important issue of motivation, deal with the teaching of letter names and sounds, and proceed to helping students read words, sentences, and paragraphs. We will end with a discussion of teaching reading comprehension.

THE FIRST STEP: MOTIVATION

The first thing a person has to have in order to gain the ability to read is the desire to do so. Because some people have been so traumatized by failure, they have become terrified of reading. Another way of saying this is that they have become print phobic. You can do several things to help students overcome this fear; the first is reading aloud. Presenting fun and interesting books in a nonthreatening way, with no demands on the student, is a first step.

Reading aloud in itself is not enough, however. Most teachers know students who love to be read to, but who freeze if *they* are asked to read. The following very particular technique is therefore recommended.

BECOMING FAMILIAR WITH THE PHYSICAL STRUCTURE OF BOOKS

Select a beautiful picture book that is age appropriate for your student. For children, a huge variety is available. For older students and adults, you can select a picture book with sophisticated illustrations, such as a folk tale. Coffee-table books such as books of photography of New England, for example, are also good choices. As you are selecting your special book, try to find one that does not have a lot of text.

Sit privately with your student and say to her something like this: "I'm going to show you a beautiful book. I'm going to give it to you now, and I want you just to open it up and look at it. But first feel how heavy it is. Check out what the binding looks like." People with dyslexia are often very attuned to the tangible world.

Therefore, helping them become comfortable with the physical nature of books is very important.

The next step is to help your student realize that there is a predictable and organized structure to published books. Help her find the title page. If appropriate, with older students, check out the dedication page and the copyright page. Discuss the purposes of these sections. Next, ask your student to leaf through the book and to enjoy the pictures. Find the end of the book and then the beginning again. Can she find the middle?

Notice if it is natural for your student to look through the book from left to right, from the beginning to the end. If this is not a natural pattern for her, show her how to do this by modeling. If she continues to have difficulty with this skill, consult your school's occupational therapist for advice. If such a professional is not available, talk with your school psychologist about the issue. A real difficulty with turning pages in a book from left to right can be an indication of a visual-motor problem that will require specific intervention.

Repeat the procedure of looking at the physical structure of books until your student seems very comfortable with picking up a picture book and looking through it. The next step is intended to help her become able to start focusing on the printed word.

Using Predictable Patterned Texts

Select several picture books with predictable patterned texts. These are books that have simple, repetitive, easily recognizable patterns. For example, in the book *The Great Big Enormous Turnip* by Alexei Tolstoy (Franklin Watts, 1968), many people and animals are involved in trying to pull up a truly enormous turnip. The language pattern of "he pulled" and "she pulled" is repeated throughout, and the illustrations also provide good clues as concerns who is doing the pulling. Students love this book and enjoy being a part of reading it over and over. You can go to your school or local library and browse through the picture book section to find other books that are appropriate.

Sit with your student and tell her that you are going to read a book together, but that she can read only one word. This approach is important, because your student probably has had many teachers trying to get her to read more text than she wished to attempt. By telling her that she can read only one word, you are telling her that the demands will not be excessive. It also can tap her sense of humor. "How come I can read only one word?" she may ask.

"Well," you can answer, "the word comes up a lot in this book, so I'll let you read it every time it's in the story—if you insist." Select words that are easily recognizable, either by meaning or form.

This technique helps students interact with print in a meaningful and enjoyable way. Often, students who have experienced failure with the written word will have developed avoidance behaviors; they will pay attention to anything but the text. Sometimes, this lack of attention is due to organic neurological factors. Emotional factors can also play a role, however, either in accentuating the original organic problem or in creating an entrenched habit of not paying attention.

Therefore, if you have a student who is really frightened of reading, take time for this work with predictable patterned text. Read your part with enthusiasm, and your student will learn to enjoy reading "her word" whenever it comes up.

THE ALPHABET: TEACHING THE SOUNDS OF ENGLISH

ASSESSMENT

Once your student has overcome her excessive fear of books and is exhibiting some interest in print, it is time to assess her knowledge of the alphabet. For reading, you primarily want to discover three things:

- Does she know the names of written letters?
- Does she know the sounds of written letters?
- Can she combine individual sounds into meaningful units?

First, ask your student to recite the alphabet to you. Notice if she tells you the alphabet, or if she just sings the alphabet song. The former is a more advanced ability than the latter. Note any missing letters or errors.

Next, refer to page 67, the quick "Alphabet Screening for Letter Names." Say to your student, "I am going to show you some letters, and I want you to tell me their names." Proceed through the list, noting any difficulties. If your student seems uncomfortable with the task, abandon it, as this is in itself very important diagnostic information. It tells you that you need to begin work at this early stage in order for your student to gain confidence.

If your student knows the names of most of the letters, go on to "Alphabet Screening for Consonant Sounds" on page 68. Tell your student that you are going to show her some letters, and you want her to tell you their sounds. Proceed through the list, recording what your student says. On letters such as "c" that have more than one sound, ask your student to tell you if she knows both sounds.

This is a short and quick diagnostic screening to get a general idea of your student's knowledge and, also, her comfort level with the sounds of English, so be sure to note any signs of nervousness or distracting behaviors that occur.

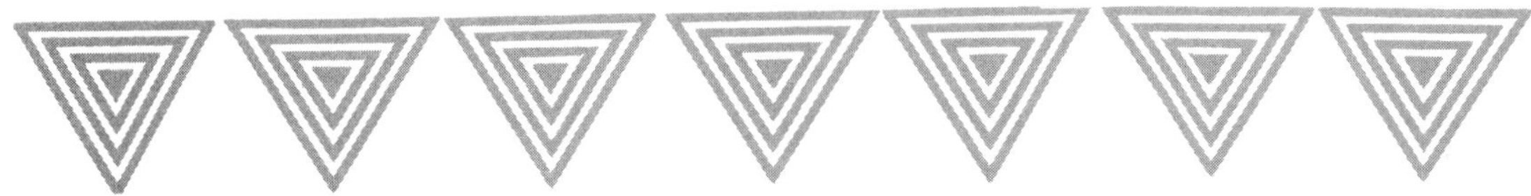

Alphabet Screening for Letter Names

LETTER	ANSWER	LETTER	ANSWER
d	______	b	______
m	______	q	______
a	______	f	______
c	______	z	______
t	______	o	______
s	______	r	______
l	______	x	______
e	______	n	______
g	______	y	______
w	______	k	______
h	______	u	______
j	______	v	______
i	______	p	______

Behavior During Testing

____

____

____

____

Name ______________________ **Date** ______________

ALPHABET SCREENING FOR CONSONANT SOUNDS

LETTER	CORRECT ANSWER
d	_____/d/
m	_____/m/
c	_____/k/ as in cat
	_____/s/ as in city
t	_____/t/
l	_____/l/
w	_____/w/
h	_____/h/
j	_____/j/
b	_____/b/
qu	_____/kw/
f	_____/f/

LETTER	CORRECT ANSWER
z	_____/z/
r	_____/r/
g	_____/g/ as in game
	_____/j/ as in gem
x	_____/ks/
n	_____/n/
v	_____/v/
s	_____/s/ as in sit
	_____/z/ as in is
p	_____/p/
k	_____/k/

Behavior During Testing

____

____

____

____

Name ______________________ **Date** ______________

General Principles for Teaching the Letter Names and Sounds of English

If your student knows the names of most letters and most individual consonant sounds, you can go on to working with books, while providing additional instruction on unfamiliar letters. If, however, your student demonstrates real discomfort or lack of knowledge of many letters, it is important to provide instruction in this area. Many books have been written on how to do this, and you may wish to refer to some of them. A book that is particularly recommended is *Developing Letter-Sound Connections: A Strategy-Oriented Alphabet Activities Program for Beginning Readers and Writers* by Cynthia Conway Waring (The Center for Applied Research in Education, 1998). This multisensory, literature-based program is very effective.

There are five basic principles for teaching the names and the sounds of the letters:

- Use multisensory instruction. Have students see, hear, say, and feel the information.
- Connect the name or sound with tangible objects. For example, when teaching the letter name for "t," you can present items such as a tack, a teddy bear, a telephone, a toothbrush and some teeth.
- Teach one letter name or sound at a time until students are comfortable with it.
- Provide frequent chances for review.
- When teaching sounds, make sure that you are presenting single sounds, as opposed to blends. In other words, teach "b" says /b/, as opposed to "bl" says /bl/.

Teaching Letter Names

Teach letter names first, if necessary. Do this by providing clear models of an individual letter and then naming the letter. Find objects in the room that begin with that letter, and write the names of the objects on the board or on a large piece of paper. Say, for example, "Look, the word 'baseball' starts with the letter 'b.'"

Usually, drawing the letter as big as possible works best. Therefore, have the student draw the letter on the board or on large paper. Let her form the letter out of strips of clay, or ask her to write it in sand. Make a tactile alphabet by cutting letters, putting glue on them, and then sprinkling sand on the glue. With permission from your student, and being sensitive to personal space concerns, you can draw the letter in the palm of her hand or on her back while you say the name. In short, provide as many opportunities as you can to connect the letter name to the student's world.

An interesting activity that students enjoy is an alphabet sequence game. Take a group of plastic letters and spray paint them one color. This helps make them look more sophisticated and, therefore, more appropriate for older students. It also takes away the distraction of the different colors.

Arrange the number of letters that is appropriate for your student in a half circle in front of her; for example, if she is just starting out, only use the "a," "b," and "c." If she is very advanced, present the whole alphabet. Then, scramble whatever number of letters are shown, and ask your student to put them in the right order. Some students particularly enjoy being timed on this task, and they like to try to beat their own time. This activity was discovered in the book *Structures and Techniques: Multisensory Teaching of Basic Language Skills* by Aylet R. Cox (Educators Publishing Service, Inc., 1984, 1980, 1977, 1975, 1974, 1969, 1967). The new edition of this book is *Foundations for Literacy: Structures and Techniques for Multisensory Teaching of Basic Written Language Skills* by Aylett Royell Cox (Educators Publishing Service, Inc. 1992).

TEACHING LETTER SOUNDS

Once a student knows most letter names, proceed to consonant sounds. These are presented before vowel sounds because short vowel sounds, especially, are often very difficult for the student with dyslexia to hear and to discriminate between. The basic technique is to provide clear and consistent models of an individual letter. Present objects that have that letter as their initial consonant sounds. For example, for the letter "b," you could show your student a basket, ball, bandage, balloon, and book. Ask your student to find objects in the room that begin with that sound. Ask her to bring objects from home (with parental permission).

With your student, decide on one object that will become the special thing that will help her remember her sound. Be very careful that the special object begins with an individual consonant, not a blend. It's also good to encourage students to select common objects.

For each sound being studied, record the letter on a 3 × 5 inch index card, and either you or your student draw a picture of the special object on the back. Practice daily with these cards. For example, your student will say "l" says /l/ as in lamp, and so on. The card deck will grow as more sounds are learned.

The frequent repetition of these sounds associated with their key words is important. Students with dyslexia often do not have good memory of relatively meaningless sound units, such as the sounds of the letters, and this is why it is essential to associate these units with meaningful objects and words.

ADDITIONAL WORK WITH LETTER SOUNDS

Some students have severe difficulty with letter sounds. These are students who forget or confuse the sounds in spite of the many multisensory opportunities they have had for learning them. They may have particular difficulty with hearing the small differences between sounds, especially vowels. They may have severe issues with phonemic awareness: in other words, identifying, knowing how many sounds are present, and knowing the order of these sounds in words. For these students, the *Lindamood*

Phoneme Sequencing Program (formerly known as the *A.D.D. Program: Auditory Discrimination in Depth*) by Charles H. Lindamood and Patricia C. Lindamood (DLM Teaching Resources, 1969, 1975, phone: 1-800-233-1819) is recommended. This program needs to be taught by a professional who has received special training. Consult with such a person, once parental permission is obtained, and describe the needs of your student. Diagnostic work may need to be done to assess whether your student needs this special remediation.

The Lindamood Phoneme Sequencing Program is a type of speech therapy program that associates the letter sounds with the tactile-kinesthetic feelings that occur in the mouth when the sounds are being produced. In addition, the program addresses the very real difficulty of sequencing and blending letter sounds. Even if some students can recognize that the word "cat" is composed of /c/ and /a/ and /t/, they can find it very difficult to combine the sounds into the word. Lindamood Phoneme Sequencing, therefore, very carefully presents techniques that will help students learn to do this.

This program requires painstaking and careful work, but it is very important that students with severe needs in the auditory discrimination area receive this type of help. If one of your students is not progressing with learning sounds at what you consider a regular rate, or is forgetting or can't seem to hear small letter differences, especially with vowels, check out this program.

READING WORDS AND SENTENCES: THE THREE CUEING SYSTEMS FOR EFFECTIVE READING

Once your student knows most individual consonant sounds, it is time to begin actual instruction with books. The teaching of the few unknown consonants and the vowel sounds can occur concurrently with the work with text. Before starting this work, however, it is important to first discuss how effective readers approach books.

To be able to read successfully, people use various cueing systems. The three main ones for figuring out how to read an individual word in a sentence are the following:

- Paying attention to the physical structure of the word; in other words, its phonetic structure
- Paying attention to meaning
- Paying attention to the grammatical structure (syntax) of written English

In the first cueing system, people often think about the initial consonant to get a sense of the identity of the word. They will notice the vowel or vowels, and will look at how long or short the word is. In the second cueing system, people think about the meaning of the sentence. If the sentence says, "The boy went to the barn to milk the (unknown word)," most students who are somewhat familiar with farm life will suspect that the last word is either "cow" or "goat." They may use their first cueing system to check out the first letter of the word. If the letter is "c," they probably will guess that the word is "cow."

The third (syntactic) cueing system can be effective in a sentence like "Jan got two new (unknown word) at the sale." The meaning cueing system is minimally effective here because Jan could have gotten many different kinds of things. The phonetic cueing system provides the information that the word has four letters and begins with "h." The student guesses that the word is "hat." This is where the third cueing system comes in, because there is something wrong with the sentence, "Jan got two new hat at the sale." It doesn't sound right. On further reflection, the student decides that because she got two of them, the word has to be "hats." When she checks the physical structure of the word, she sees an "s" at the end of it and makes her final decision: The word is "hats."

Successful readers use a combination of all three cueing systems, and the main goal of beginning reading instruction is to help students develop a nice balance of using all three. Too much attention to the phonetic structure of words encourages students not to think about the general idea of what they are reading. Too much emphasis on meaning cues, with no attention to the physical structure of words, doesn't help in situations where meaning is not obvious, and it encourages wild guessing. Students can really use the third cueing system only if they can already read most of the words in a sentence, so it is not effective if used by itself for beginning readers.

You need to have your students do three things when they face unfamiliar text:

- Look at the words.
- Think about what they are reading.
- Listen to how the sentences sound.

THE FIRST CUEING SYSTEM—PHONICS

Most people have never been given information about the structure of the English language and thus they fear that it is too complex to be of any use to beginning readers. On the contrary, the English language is based on a few simple principles:

- Letters refer to specific sounds.
- Individual words are composed of one or more units of sound called syllables.
- Many words are borrowed from other languages, and these can be unique in their pronunciation and spelling.

It is true that English can be confusing. For example, one letter can refer to more than one sound, as when "c" can say /k/ or /s/. Furthermore, a given sound can be spelled by more than one letter combination, as when /f/ is represented by either "f" or "ph." And then there are all the words that are exactly the same, but have completely different meanings, like the word "left." This word can be an adjective to represent a certain side of the body such as our *left* hand, or a verb telling that a person has *left* a room, or a noun describing the political *left*.

The vagaries of English are many, especially because so many words have been borrowed from other languages. For the purpose of teaching beginning reading, however, two principles should be remembered:

- Keep it simple.
- Present only high-utility phonetic concepts.

When approached in this way, learning phonics can give students a valuable tool when facing a new word. They don't have to be experts, they just need a sense that most words—85 percent to be exact—have a logical structure to their physical makeup.

What Is the Structure of the English Language?

The following is a brief overview of the structure of English. Becoming familiar with this structure will help you feel more comfortable with phonics instruction.

- There are 21 consonants. These letters represent units of sound that usually end quickly, such as in "p" and "t." Consonants such as "m" and "l" can be continued with the voice, but the mouth is generally closed.
- There are combinations of consonants that can have unique sounds, such as "sh," which represents /sh/; "ch," which represents /ch/; "ph," which represents /f/; and "th," which represents /th/.
- There are 6 vowels: "a," "i," "o," "u," "e," and sometimes "y." These letters represent sounds that can go on indefinitely, limited only by the amount of breath a person has. The mouth is usually open. Vowels can be pronounced long: "i" says its name as in "hi." Vowels can also be short, as when "i" says /i/ as in "him." The vowel "y" can say long /e/ as in "penny," or short /i/ as in "gym."
- Several combinations of vowels represent unique sounds; for example, "oo" represents the /oo/ sound, as in "moon."
- Several combinations of consonant and vowels represent unique sounds; "ing," represents the /ing/ sound as in "king."
- Words are composed of units of sounds called syllables. Syllables each have at least one vowel and varying combinations of other letters. There are seven types of syllables in the English language:

  1. *Closed syllable:* A single vowel is closed in or stopped by a consonant, as in "it," and "cat."

2. *Open syllable:* A single vowel is not followed by a consonant, and thus the mouth could conceivably stay open. Two examples of open syllables are "go" and "me."
3. *Vowel-consonant-e:* A vowel is followed by one consonant, which is immediately followed by an "e." In this type of syllable, the vowel is long, as in "ate."
4. *Vowel combination syllable:* Two vowels combine to make one sound, as when "ai" says long /a/ as in "rain."
5. *R-controlled syllable:* The letter "r" exerts its powerful influence on any vowel that it follows. For example, the "a" is neither short nor long when it is followed by an "r" in the word "car."
6. *Final syllable:* This is a unique and frequently occurring combination of letters that is seen only at the end of multisyllabic words. Two examples are "tle," as in "turtle," and "tion" as in "mention."
7. *Letter-team syllable:* This is a highly visible and common group of letters that always make the same sound, either alone or in combination with other letters. Two examples are "ing," as in "ring," and "old," as in "told."

It is important for you to have a basic understanding of this structure. For your beginning reader, however, you need only start presenting frequently used letters and letter combinations. They don't need an overall understanding at this point.

How to Teach the First Cueing System

As we look at how to provide effective instruction for phonics, we can look back at the Orton-Gillingham program, which provides an excellent model. Common elements present in many lessons of the Orton-Gillingham type are as follows:

- ***Flash Card Drill.*** Students have individual card packs that contain the letters and sounds they have already studied. As new sounds are introduced, new cards are added. Each card will have the letter and either a picture or a written model of the key word for the sound of the letter being studied. Key words are words that the student memorizes to help her remember the particular sound associated with the letter. For example, for the short vowel "a," a frequently used key word is "apple." The card for this sound, therefore, will have the letter "a" written on one side, and either a picture of an apple or the word "apple" written on the back. While practicing with his card deck, the student will say "a" says /a/ as in "apple." In every lesson, students practice with their card decks, thus providing important reinforcement.
- ***Word List Reading.*** A list of phonetically regular words, all containing a particular letter-sound combination being studied is shown to the student. She reads the individual words in the list.

- ***Sentence Reading and Reading in Context.*** An effort is made to find text that contains only phonetic elements that the student has studied. The student then reads this text.
- ***Studying Sounds.*** The teacher says a sound, and the student writes the letter that represents it. The usual number of sounds presented is eight.
- ***Spelling, or Encoding.*** The teacher says a word and the student writes it. All words will contain only letters and sounds for which the student has received careful instruction. All of these words will be phonetically regular. Approximately five to ten words will be presented.
- ***Dictation.*** The teacher dictates a sentence or more, and the student writes them. All of the words in the sentence will be phonetically regular and will contain elements with which the student is familiar. If phonetically irregular words are included, models are provided unless it is known that the student has memorized the word.

To summarize, a lesson will probably include work with the card deck, some practice reading individual words that contain the element being studied, and a good amount of reading in context. At some point in the lesson, the student will also write letters that represent sounds, and words and sentences that contain phonetic elements that she has studied.

The one remaining issue is the most effective sequence for introducing phonetic elements. Most programs of the Orton-Gillingham type begin with the short vowels. As an example, the Wilson Reading System, a program developed by Barbara A. Wilson especially for adolescents and adults, first presents a few consonants and then all five short vowels. Some letter teams are introduced, for example, "ing" and "ink," and then vowel-consonant-e syllables are presented. To obtain specific information about this sequence, contact:

WILSON READING SYSTEM
Wilson Language Training Corporation
162 West Main St.
Milbury, MA 01527-1943
508-865-5699

INTEGRATING THE THREE CUEING SYSTEMS

The following approach is recommended for helping students achieve a nice balance of the three cueing systems. It is particularly effective because it integrates elements of both Orton-Gillingham and whole-language philosophies.

This approach is taken from the book *Developing Independent Readers: Strategy-Oriented Reading Activities for Learners with Special Needs* by Cynthia

Conway Waring (The Center for Applied Research in Education, 1995). Its sequence of phonetic elements is unique, beginning with the high utility letter-team "ing." The vowel-combination syllable "oo" is next introduced, and then the open syllables with all five vowels. Waring's book contains much more specific information on the techniques summarized here. It also provides 34 literature-based units that give detailed directions for planning and presenting lessons. Even though the literature cited is primarily of the picture-book variety, the sequence and techniques of the program can be used with older students. Books that contain photographs and limited text, for example, can even be used with adults.

This program outlines four stages of reading instruction:

- Listening to a teacher read a book
- Oral cloze reading
- Supported reading
- Independent reading

THE FIRST STAGE: LISTENING TO A TEACHER READ A BOOK

This is very similar to, but different from the read-aloud technique used for helping students overcome print phobia. You are doing the same basic thing—reading a book out loud to your students—but your focus is different. When reading aloud to help heal print phobia, you are primarily thinking about emotional issues. You are asking yourself questions like "Is my student enjoying the book? Is she touching it readily and looking at the pictures? Is she engaged in what we are doing?"

When you are reading aloud for the first stage of more formal reading instruction, as outlined in Waring's book, you are planning ahead for when your student will be reading the words. Thus, you are modeling the following important strategies:

Preview the book. Together with your student, physically examine the book, especially the pictures. You are detectives, looking for clues as to what the book may be about.

Talk about what the text is saying. Asking questions of your student about the story line, the characters, and the plot encourages her to relate what she hears in the spoken words to what she thinks and feels in her own life.

Predict and check what the text is saying. This discussion also promotes the use of your student's good common sense as she reads—and it's a lot of fun to see if you can predict how the plot is going to turn out.

Examine unfamiliar vocabulary. You can do this lightly, saying, "Well, let's see if we can figure out what that word means from the rest of the sentence." Here, you are modeling using meaning clues. Use this cueing system when it will have a good chance of being effective for a given word. Otherwise, just lightly tell your student what the unfamiliar word means.

Once you are reading to your student, begin to delete occasional words that she will easily be able to provide from listening to the story. Do this only when it will not interfere with the enjoyment of the book. At first, omit highly predictable words at the ends of sentences, especially rhymes or words that are repeated in patterns. Then, once your student is very comfortable with that, omit important nouns and verbs that are easily predicted from meaning cues. Your student is not looking at the text at this point. She is looking only at the pictures. She is exclusively using meaning cues for her predictions.

THE SECOND STAGE: ORAL CLOZE READING

The term *cloze* was introduced by W. Taylor in his article "Cloze Procedure: A New Tool for Measuring Readability" (*Journalism Quarterly*, 1953, 30, 415-433). It is taken from the Gestalt concept of being able to cloze, or fill in, something that is incomplete by using prior knowledge.

In Waring's second stage of reading instruction, students begin actually to look at the text. You point to the words as you continue to read aloud, and the student follows along. This is where you begin to teach the integration of the three cueing systems of thinking about what is read, looking at the physical structure of words, and listening to sentences.

Together, you preview the book. Then, say that you are going to ask for some help with reading. When you pause, you'd like the student to say what the word might be. At first, omit highly recognizable sight words such as "I" and "is." It's a good idea to start with one or two, and then increase the number as your student feels happy with the task.

Next, follow the same pattern as in the read-aloud technique: Delete highly predictable rhyming words or repeated words in patterns, and then move on to nouns and verbs with obvious meaning. At first, delete words at the ends of sentences, as this is easiest. All of the meaning and grammatical cues of the sentence have already been read. Then, when your student can be successful, eliminate words in the middle or even beginnings of sentences. This will help model the need for the strategy of moving on and reading the rest of the sentence in order to gain information about an unknown word.

At this stage, it is helpful to do supplementary work with the cloze method apart from the reading of books. An activity sheet, "Cloze Sentences with Short 'a' as in 'Ran,'" which illustrates the use of the cloze method in combination with the instruction of phonetic structure is provided on page 78. This activity should be done with the teacher supporting the reading.

Cloze Sentences with Short "a" as in "Ran"

Choose words from the word list to finish the sentences.

1. "I am not lost," said Latoya, "because I have a ________________."
2. It is fun to run barefoot in the ________________.
3. If you want more light, turn on the ________________.
4. To be mailed, the letter needs a ________________.
5. The ________________ of the U.S.A. is red, white, and blue.
6. A ________________ shell can be found in the ocean.

WORD LIST

clam	stamp
sand	flag
lamp	map

Name ______________________________ **Date** ____________________

A Note on Teaching Multisyllabic Words. Spend a lot of time on single-syllable words with the cloze method, until your students are very comfortable with this technique. As you are reading books, however, model breaking down large words into smaller units by using your thumb to cover parts of words, such as obvious endings, and halves of compound words. As you proceed, begin to cover the second syllable in a multisyllabic word, and move your thumb to reveal each new syllable as the word is read. In the very beginning of instruction, this can be done informally with an easy manner. For example, you can say something like, "Oh look, when I cover the 'ing' in 'going,' the little word 'go' is left."

After your student is very familiar with your modeling in this way, take a word from the text and write it down. Make sure that the student understands the concepts of syllables, vowels, and consonants. Tell her that you are going to underline the vowels in the word and draw a circle around the consonants.

Tell your student that when she is looking at an unfamiliar long word, she has to make an important decision, and that is whether the underlined vowels are going to be short or long. Sometimes, two vowels are together and they make a special sound, but you will be there to help your student with those kinds of syllables.

As we get back to this important decision of whether a vowel standing alone is short or long, there are strategies to help readers decide about this. The following is a short summary:

> ***Strategy One-One Consonant:*** If there is one consonant separating vowels in a word, divide first before the consonant, as in "Chi-na." The first vowel is then long. If the word does not make sense, as in "li-mit," divide after the consonant, making "lim-it."
>
> ***Strategy Two-Two Consonants:*** First, try dividing between the two consonants, as in "muf-fin." If the word does not make sense, as in "neg-lect," divide before the two consonants, making "ne-glect."
>
> ***Strategy Three-Three Consonants:*** First, try dividing after the first consonant, as in the word "or-chard." If that does not work, as in the word "tran-sfer," divide after the second consonant sound. The word "trans-fer" is then read.

It is important that this work not feel intimidating to students. Tell your students that they are going to have to use their good detective skills to make these new words say what they are. Present only words that are obvious and easy in the beginning. As their confidence grows, your students will enjoy breaking down large words into smaller units. An activity sheet, "Cloze Sentences with Multisyllabic Words with I-Consonant-E (as in "pine"), is provided on page 80. This activity should be done with the teacher supporting the reading.

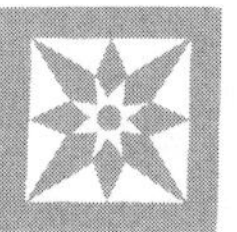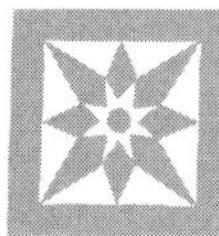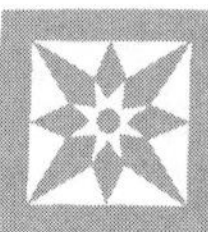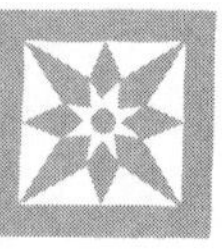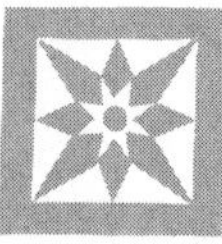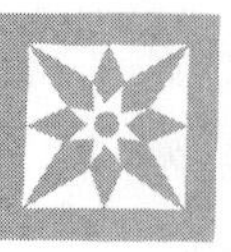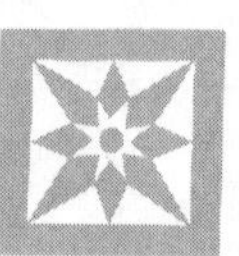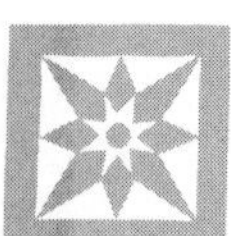

CLOZE SENTENCES WITH MULTISYLLABIC WORDS WITH I-CONSONANT-E (AS IN "PINE")

Choose words from the word list to finish the sentences.

1. Juan and Jim sat around the ________________ and told stories.
2. The ________________ said that the batter was out.
3. "I want to ________________ you to my party," said Kim.
4. You can get burned if you stay in the ________________ too long.
5. "I ________________ that beautiful painting," Malcolm said.
6. Sarah went ________________ the cabin to get out of the rain.

WORD LIST

umpire	invite
admire	campfire
inside	sunshine

Name ________________________________ **Date** ________________

The Third Stage: Supported Reading

According to Waring, it is time to move on to this next stage of reading when

- your student is competent and comfortable with the cloze method,
- she has her own collection of sight words that she easily recognizes in text, and
- she knows sufficient phonetic elements, such as most consonant sounds and many vowels.

In this stage, the student does all the reading of the text, and you support the use of appropriate strategies. If your student begins this next stage and appears largely uncomfortable, immediately return to the prior stage. Make this transition with as little attention given to it as possible, so your student does not see it as a failure.

Some very important things happen at the Supported Reading stage. One of the most important is that the student points to the words she is reading, as opposed to having you do so. Some students don't want to point, and some teachers have been taught that this physical act can inhibit fluency. With students with dyslexia, however, pointing to the words helps them maintain their attention and focus on their reading. It is an important technique that needs to be encouraged at this stage.

Carefully choose texts that are well within the student's ability to read. Keep the amount of time given for this reading well within student's capacities. You want your student to work hard, but you don't want her to be exhausted or overwhelmed. Thus, she can begin to see reading as an enjoyable challenge, instead of a dreadful task.

Your job as a teacher at this stage is to give your student plenty of safe and quiet time in which to interact with text, to give clues as she faces words that are difficult for her, and to help her learn the important habit of self-correcting when she has incorrectly read a word. As much as possible, give nonverbal clues. If the word is "down," for example, point down to the floor. If the word is illustrated in the text, point to the picture. The use of nonverbal cues helps maintain the nice flow of reading without too many teacher-words interrupting.

You do need to keep a theoretical framework in mind as you give these clues. Your goal is to give meaning clues first, syntactic clues second, and phonetic clues last.

Two examples of meaning clues are as follows:

> "What kind of animal do you think would live in the ocean?"
>
> "That word is the opposite of _______ ."

To give syntactic cues, first reread the passage so that your student can hear the flow of the language. Then, ask questions like the following:

> "Did that word sound right there?"
>
> "Do people really talk like that?"
>
> "I thought that there was more than one cat in the story."

For phonetic clues, say things like these examples:

"Oh, I see a 't' at the beginning of that word."

"It's got that 'ai,' as in 'rain.'"

"Check out the ending."

As your student progresses, give fewer clues and more time for her to be independent with her reading. Possibly the most important purpose of your clues is to model the types of cueing systems that can be used. Ultimately, you want your student to be able to give clues to herself.

Your goal is to help your student integrate the three cueing systems, so that she can have three powerful tools with which to read. It's critically important that you give her plenty of time to think and analyze. All too often, teachers feel that they aren't doing their job if they are not constantly informing or instructing. It feels too restful to sit quietly while a student takes time to think about what a word could be, but this is what your student needs most. Think of your job as being the guardian of the quiet time.

When reading is done in pairs of students or with larger groups, three important rules need to be observed:

1. Every reader is given comfortable, safe time for thinking.
2. No one offers clues unless the reader asks for them.
3. Clues are given in this order: meaning first, sentence structure next, and phonetic clues last.

Even small children can be taught to observe these rules, thus a safe environment is created in which all students can practice their reading.

THE FOURTH STAGE: INDEPENDENT READING

It is a judgment call exactly when students arrive at this advanced stage, but often you will see your student independently pick up a book from a table or shelf and begin to look through it. She is now using all three cueing systems in a balanced and effective way, and she is ready emotionally to move on.

Here, your job is to provide good books that will offer appropriate challenge. The following are good resources to help you find such books:

- *Books Children Love: A Guide to the Best Children's Literature* by Elizabeth Wilson, Foreword by Susan Schaeffer Macaulay (Crossway Books, 1987).
- *The New York Times Parent's Guide to the Best Books for Children* by Eden Ross Lipson, children's book editor of *The New York Times* (Times Books, 1991).
- *Books to build On: A Grade-by-Grade Resource Guide for Parents and Teachers*, edited by John Holdren and E. D. Hirsch, Jr. (Delta, 1996).

- *Reading Rainbow Guide to Children's Books: The 101 Best Titles* by Twila Liggett, Ph.D., and Cynthia Mayer Benfield, with an introduction by LeVar Burton (A Citadel Press Book, published by Carol Publishing Group, 1994, 1996).

Once you have gotten a good book into the hands of your student, sit with her and provide silent support. When she looks to you to provide clues for a difficult word, either nod or smile. She will soon learn that you aren't going to give her specific help, because she can now use her cueing systems and figure out the word for herself.

There are specific things that you can do, however, at this stage to encourage further progress. Teach and model the following strategies:

- previewing books
- retelling
- review reading
- anticipating meaning
- reading on
- rereading
- cross-checking
- self-correcting

These strategies are presented at earlier stages, but they are more focused upon here. Students have been practicing using a balance of cueing systems as they look at an individual word. Now, they need to look to the whole body of text to help them find meaning.

Let us look at each of these strategies more closely. Previewing books is self-explanatory. With your student, physically look at the book—its cover and any illustrations. Read the information presented on the book jacket flaps.

Once a student has read a certain amount of text, ask her to retell what has happened. This can occur during a reading session or on consecutive days.

In review reading, ask your student to reread some text. This reminds her of what the book is about, and supports the idea that good readers go back and reread, either for pleasure, or for information, or to figure out where they are in the story.

Anticipating meaning is similar to what is done when you preview books, but it's done on a more specific scale. Does the chapter take place, for example, on a city street? Well, then there may be lots of words about cities in the text. Does a certain character seem angry? He may express this in some way.

In reading on, if a student comes to a word that she absolutely does not know, she can either pause at that word or say "blank" and then go on and read the rest of the sentence. In this way, she may get more meaning clues to use.

She can also reread a certain part of the passage. If reading on has not helped, she can start from the beginning of the sentence or paragraph and try again.

Cross-checking is very important. Here, the reader may make a guess about a word strictly from meaning. For example, the sentence could read, "Harry went to the __________ to buy eggs." The reader guesses that the word is "store." So she asks herself, "Does 'store' sound right in the sentence?" Yes, it does. But the word could be "farm," because sometimes people actually go to farms to buy eggs. So the reader asks herself, "What letter does the word start with? Ah, an 's,' so the word probably is 'store.'" If the word had begun with an "f," the reader would then have used another good technique—self-correction.

HOW TO TEACH READING COMPREHENSION

Students have already been working on reading comprehension as they have been learning to decode words and sentences. When you help them to focus on the meaning of text and, in fact, to use this as a cueing system to predict unfamiliar words, you have already begun the process for good comprehension. As they approach more complex texts and longer stories, however, reading comprehension needs to be focused upon.

WHAT DO STUDENTS WITH DYSLEXIA NEED?

Students with dyslexia sometimes need structured work as they confront more difficult text. As you plan this instruction, keep in mind the following learning styles that are characteristic of people with dyslexia:

- They like to be actively involved in learning; in other words, participatory instruction is best.
- They learn well through multimodality approaches.
- They often are interested in the physical structure of things, and graphic two- and three-dimensional forms help them become organized.
- They can have limited attention spans and high activity levels.

THE BEST GENERAL APPROACH

The book *Dyslexia: Research and Resource Guide* by Carol Sullivan Spafford and George S. Grosser (Allyn and Bacon, 1996)* presents an excellent summary of what is needed for an effective program in this area. Students need

- A purpose for reading

---

*A summary from *Dyslexia: Research and Resource Guide* by Carol Sullivan Spafford and George S. Grosser (Allyn and Bacon, 1996). Used by permission.

- Acknowledgment and discussion of preexisting knowledge that they may have about the subject of the text
- Discussion of the main ideas and/or characters
- Modeling of questions effective readers ask about the text as they are reading
- Modeling of questions effective readers ask about the reading process they are using with the text
- Writing activities that will integrate the knowledge or impressions gained from the text

To establish a purpose, previewing sets the stage. Readers gain a broad sense of what they will be encountering. Because students with dyslexia often have such developed senses of physical structure, it is helpful to look at the whole section to be read. Are there pictures that will be informative? Are there main headings or summary sections? How long is the piece? All of these queries take away some of the mystique and, thus, the fear of the work.

Another critically important aspect of setting a purpose is motivation. Students with dyslexia do much better if they are interested in the subject, whether it is fiction or nonfiction. This is an important factor to discover about your student, and time spent in the process is well used. Does your student prefer stories, and what type? Mysteries? Humor? If she prefers to read to gain information, what particular subjects appeal to her the most? Space? Basketball? As much as possible, select reading material that is interesting to your students. As they become more capable readers, they will learn to handle text that is less interesting to them. Three Interest Inventories are provided on pages 86–88. "What I Like to Read" is for the elementary level, "My Reading Interests" is for intermediate level, and "An Interest Inventory for Reading" is for secondary to adult.

The second important part of a good reading comprehension program is helping students recall preexisting relevant information. Here again, especially for early instruction in this area, try to select subject matter about which students have a good deal of prior knowledge. Is the story, for example, set in Canada? Has the student visited that country? Is the paragraph about stars? Has the student ever visited a planetarium? Time spent discussing the topic will set the stage for the actual reading, and as your student faces the brand new text, she will feel that she is looking at something familiar.

Discussing the main themes, ideas, characters, and important details in the text is the third important thing to do. Teachers tend to do this with all students, regardless of their learning style. Students with dyslexia need lots of this interaction.

Effective readers ask themselves questions about the content as they read—questions like "What are the names of the planets in our galaxy? Will I learn them on this page?" This is the fourth aspect of a good program. To ask questions, a reader has to be actively involved with the text, and this is not something that comes naturally to all students. That is why it is most helpful for you to model the process *you* might go through. Talk out loud. Express your thoughts and questions. Then, gently help your students to do the same. As they gain practice, they will begin to ask themselves questions silently as they read.

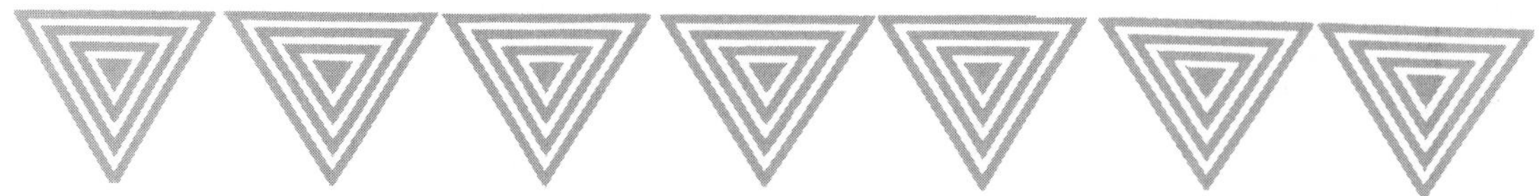

What I Like to Read

Put a checkmark on whatever is true for you.

1. I like books with:
   - only pictures _____
   - lots of pictures _____
   - some pictures _____
   - only words _____
2. I like books that:
   - help me learn things _____
   - tell me stories _____
3. I like books that:
   - deal with serious subjects _____
   - make me laugh _____
   - have poems _____
   - have riddles and jokes _____
4. In fiction, I like:
   - adventures _____
   - fantasies _____
   - folk tales and fables _____
   - mysteries _____
   - science fiction _____
   - stories about kids in real-life situations _____
   - stories about animals _____
   - stories about people in the past _____
   - stories about events in the past _____
5. In nonfiction, I like to read about:

animals	_____	history	_____
art	_____	math	_____
challenging situations	_____	music	_____
crafts and hobbies	_____	science	_____
famous people	_____	sports	_____

Here are some other things I like to read about:

____

Name ______________________________ **Date** ________________

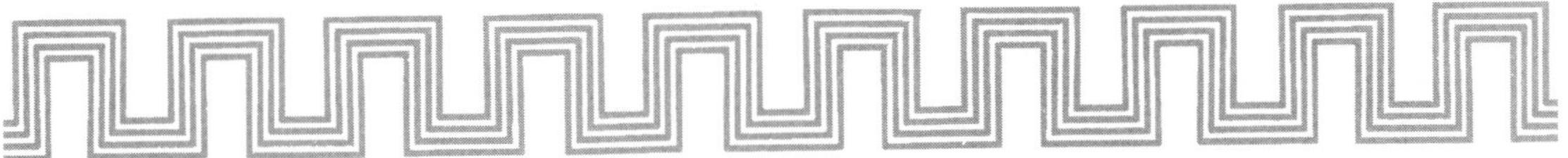

My Reading Interests

Put a checkmark on whatever is true for you.

1. I like books with:
   - lots of pictures _____
   - large print _____
   - a few, short chapters _____
   - long chapters _____
2. I like:
   - fiction _____
   - nonfiction _____
   - books of poetry _____
   - fables and folktales _____
3. In fiction, I enjoy:
   - fantasy _____
   - historical fiction _____
   - humor _____
   - mystery _____
   - realistic stories about people _____
   - realistic stories about animals _____
   - science fiction _____
4. In non-fiction, I like to read about:
   - animals _____
   - autobiography _____
   - art _____
   - biography _____
   - challenging situations _____
   - crafts and hobbies _____
   - famous people _____
   - history _____
   - math _____
   - music _____
   - science _____
   - sports _____

Here are some other things I like to read about:

____

This is a book that I have really enjoyed:

____

Name ____________________________ **Date** _________________

AN INTEREST INVENTORY FOR READING

Put a checkmark on whatever is true for you.

1. I enjoy books with:
   - some pictures _____
   - large print _____
   - short chapters _____
   - long chapters _____
2. I like:
   - fiction _____
   - nonfiction _____
   - essays _____
   - personal journals _____
   - books of poetry _____
   - magazines _____
   - newspapers _____
3. In fiction, I enjoy:
   - fantasy _____
   - historical fiction _____
   - humor _____
   - mystery _____
   - realistic stories about people _____
   - romance novels _____
   - science fiction _____
   - westerns _____
4. In nonfiction, I like to read about:
   - animals _____
   - art _____
   - autobiography _____
   - biography _____
   - challenging situations _____
   - contemporary moral issues _____
   - contemporary political issues _____
   - crafts and hobbies _____
   - famous people _____
   - history _____
   - math _____
   - music _____
   - science _____
   - sports _____

Here are some other things I enjoy reading about:

____

Name ______________________________ **Date** ____________________

The fifth important aspect of a good reading comprehension program is to help students ask themselves questions about the reading process itself. They can ask themselves, for example, "Am I understanding what I am reading? Do I need to slow down or reread because this part is so hard?" Here again, teacher modeling is very important. As you regularly and repeatedly vocalize the questioning process you might use, your students will hear what is possible.

The last component of a good reading comprehension program is to integrate writing. Some people are surprised at this, because the act of writing is in itself difficult for many students with dyslexia. This is a good example, however, of where integration of curriculum can be very effective. As students write about what they read, or as they use information from text in creative writing projects, the back-and-forth nature of reading and writing causes them to feed each other. Students with dyslexia need to be actively involved with their subject matter. Writing is a very potent way of helping them become involved with text.

The two independent activity sheets "A Cinderella List" and "A Special Letter," on pages 92 and 94 illustrate the integration of reading and writing. You can also refer to Chapter 9, "Teaching Writing" for other suggestions on how to help students use this valuable skill.

Activities for Reading Comprehension

General guidelines have been offered up to this point. A few specific activities are presented here:

1. ***Self-sustained Silent Reading.*** Students need a great deal of practice with reading comprehension. The act of simply reading provides some of this, and for this reason, periods of time during the school day when students can sit quietly and just read are very valuable. This technique has been formalized into a system called self-sustained silent reading. Here, students and teachers and, in fact, all adults at the school, set aside a certain block of time each day to enjoy a book. This technique is very valuable. Even if students are not yet independent readers, they can look through a wordless picture book or examine a book of photographs. The atmosphere of relaxation and rest helps students overcome any lingering feelings of discomfort, and thus they will be able to use more of their whole selves to understand what they are reading. Teachers can model their good relationships with books and discuss their understandings of what they have been reading at the end of the silent reading time.

2. ***Photocopy and Preview.*** This is a previewing activity. Because students with dyslexia are often so graphically oriented, it helps them to have information presented two-dimensionally. Photocopy a page of nonfiction text that contains headings, boldface type, and other print styles that indicate important aspects of text. With your students, highlight these important markers and discuss what they mean.

3. ***Make a "What I Know" Poster.*** This activity focuses on background information. Have your students draw or make a collage of what they already know about a subject that they will read about. Advanced students can write phrases or sentences about their knowledge on a piece of drawing paper.

4. ***Photocopy and Highlight Main Ideas.*** This activity helps students discover the main idea. Photocopy a page of text. With your students, discuss what the main ideas are in the paragraphs shown, and ask them to highlight these sentences.

5. ***Speed-read Easy Text.*** This activity helps students recognize main ideas. Select text that is well below your student's comfortable reading level. Tell her that you know that she can read this easily, but that she is going to practice with it so that reading harder text becomes easier. Ask her to read a paragraph, and as soon as she has finished, to tell you about it. Tell her that speed is important, and that she should tell you only about the important things she has learned.

6. ***Illustrate a Concept or Draw Two Scenes in a Story.*** This activity also focuses on finding the main idea. For nonfiction work, ask students to select and draw a picture that illustrates an important concept. For fiction, take a piece of drawing paper and fold it in half. Ask students to draw two scenes in the story that occur sequentially.

7. ***In Textbooks, Look at the Questions at the Ends of Chapters.*** This activity teaches questioning skills, in addition to being a good previewing technique. Sometimes, students think they are cheating if they look ahead at the questions, and they feel very relieved and happy to learn that it is a good idea to do so. As an additional part of this activity, students can, once they have read the text, write questions of their own that they feel are better than the presented ones.

8. ***Keep a "This is How I Feel About Reading" Journal.*** This activity helps students become reflective about their own reading process. Model good entries, such as "I like reading about bugs," or "The story I'm reading has lots of characters, so I'm going to keep a list of them to keep them straight." The journal writing should be simple and easy and fun. If students seem uncomfortable with it after an introductory period, abandon the project. An independent activity sheet, "This Is How I Feel About Reading," is provided on page 91. It models one possibility for a journal of this type.

9. ***Write a List.*** This activity integrates writing and reading. Use whatever you are reading to inspire a list idea. Are you reading about birds, for example? Students can write a list of things that fly. Of course, they are allowed to include the birds that are mentioned in the text. An independent activity sheet, "A Cinderella List," which illustrates the use of this activity with a folk tale, is provided on page 92.

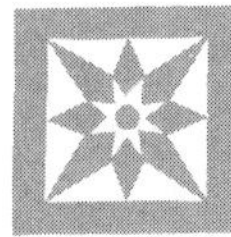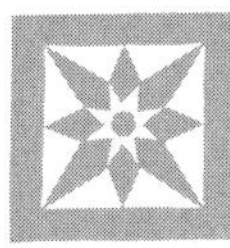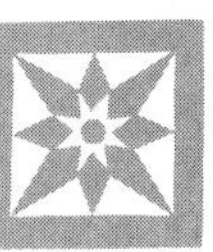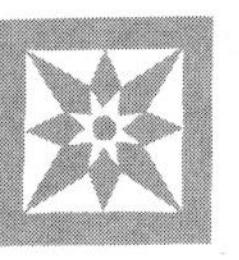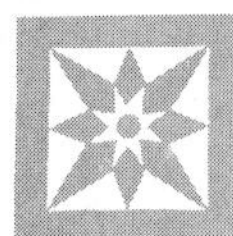

THIS IS HOW I FEEL ABOUT READING

Today, I read the book ____

I read this many pages: ____________

In terms of difficulty, the reading was:

____

In terms of how much I was interested in the book, the reading was:

____

In terms of how much I understood what I was reading, I:

____

To be an effective reader, I think I should: (check what applies)

- slow down _____
- read more carefully _____
- ask for some help from my teacher _____
- discuss what I'm reading with a friend _____
- read just like I've been doing _____

In general, I think that reading this book is:

____

____

____

____

Name ________________________________ **Date** __________________

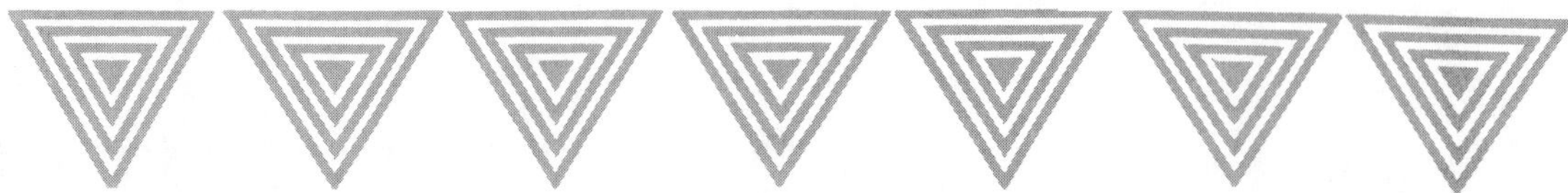

A CINDERELLA LIST

With your teacher, read the story Cinderella. Notice the things that Cinderella's fairy godmother gave her, like a new fancy dress and glass slippers. Then, make a list of the things you would ask for if you had a fairy godmother.

Name ______________________________ **Date** ________________

10. ***Paraphrase a Paragraph of Nonfiction Text.*** This activity integrates writing and reading. Ask your student to read a given paragraph, and then to write it herself as if she were teaching the information it contained to a much younger student. Encourage your student to write a topic sentence, a few sentences that give details, and an ending summary sentence.

11. ***Write a letter from a character.*** This activity also integrates writing and reading. Ask your student to select a character from a story she is reading. She will then pretend to be that character and write a letter to herself. The character can either write about a particular scene or about what has happened in the whole book. An independent activity sheet for this activity, "A Special Letter," is provided on page 94.

What to Do if There Are Severe Problems with Reading Comprehension

If students do not respond to activities such as the ones listed above, they may need specialized help in this area. One program that can be very helpful is outlined in *Visualizing and Verbalizing for Language Comprehension and Thinking* by Nanci Bell (Nancibell, Inc., 1991). The basic premise of this program is that people must be able to create visual pictures in their minds in order to understand spoken as well as written language. Through a very specific sequence of instruction, students who have difficulty in this area are taught to create these mental pictures. Special and careful study by the teacher is required, but *Visualizing and Verbalizing* gives the information on how to provide this instruction. If you have a student who has significant needs in this cognitive area, you may wish to learn to use this program.

Other Helpful Programs

Reading Stories for Comprehension Success: 45 High-Interest Lessons with Reproducible Selections and Questions That Make Kids Think by Katherine L. Hall (vol. 1: Primary Level, Grades 1-3, vol. 2: Intermediate Level, Grades 4-6, The Center for Applied Research in Education, 1996) provides interesting selections for students to read. Each lesson suggests related activities, books, CDs, and videos. This program is difficult for the very beginning reader. For others more advanced, however, it offers text that students will enjoy reading, and it also gives suggestions on how to create background knowledge and related thinking with regard to each selection. The richness of this program is illustrative of a good reading comprehension program.

A Special Letter

Choose a favorite character from the book you are reading. Pretend to be that person and write a letter back to yourself.

If, for example, you are pretending to be Anne Frank, the young Jewish girl who hid from the Nazis, you could start your letter this way:

Dear Jason,

You live in such a different world from mine, and I am glad of it. But let me tell you a little about me and my family.

Dear ________________,

____

____

____

____

____

____

____

____

Name ______________________________ **Date** ________________

The Kim Marshall Series: Reading, Books 1 and 2 by Kim Marshall (Educators Publishing Service, Inc., 1984, 1982) consists of two books, each of which contains over 90 stories. These are mostly about interesting real-life happenings, such as the Watergate break-in, and about people, such as the story of Cicely Tyson. Each story has several reading comprehension questions. These books are particularly helpful because of the high motivation level of all of the stories. Students are interested in them and often want to discuss the information at great length.

Rereading for Understanding by Thelma Gwinn Thurstone (Science Research Associates, Inc., 1978, 1965, 1963) provides a series of cards that are carefully sequenced in terms of level of difficulty. Each card has several short reading selections and questions with multiple choice answers. This program provides good practice for those students who enjoy doing it.

Reading Comprehension in Varied Subject Matter by Jane Ervin (Educators Publishing Service, Inc., 1970-1993) is a series of books that provide practice in reading comprehension from grade 2 to junior high and up. Each lesson has a selection for students to read. They then answer questions about the main idea, important details, sequencing, inferential understanding, and vocabulary. These books are good for supervised independent work.

INTERVIEW WITH MIKE

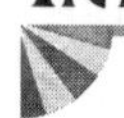

Mike is a paramedic who works for a fire department. He also runs his own construction company. After receiving appropriate instruction as an adult, he now reads to gain information and for enjoyment. Mike often prefers to read rather than to watch TV. He particularly enjoys historical fiction.

What was reading like for you in elementary school?

Hard. I dreaded it. Again, you know, I couldn't focus on it, and I really needed to do that. One thing that stuck in my mind: Brenda, a real smart girl. She used to read to the class. And me, I always thought there'd be someone out there to do that for me.

The thing is, I always had to have a reason to do something, you know. Math, I could see what it was, but I had a hard time with reading. I didn't realize I needed to read. That was my rationale. I've always been good in math. I could never put that same effort into reading.

What did you do in your summer program?

(Mike was sent to a special summer school for several summers when he was in elementary school.)

One thing we had to do was read in class. I dreaded going there. It put you right on the spot. We had to read a page. You were assigned to read a page, and as long as it took, you had to read that page. I used to find all kinds of reasons for not going, but . . . I'm still in touch with one of the guys I rode down with. He gave up. He never made it through high school.

What about junior high?

It was still hard getting through it. I got into social studies and stuff like that where there was a lot of reading involved.

What was hard about reading in junior high?

Understanding, pronouncing the words. When somebody read to me, I could understand it, but if I was trying to read it, if I came to a hard word, I wound up skipping over it and nothing made sense after that. I was skipping over too much. The easy stuff I could do, but when we got into names . . . Peoples' names, I always used to skip. Towns, stuff like that. The longer words.

What did you do to avoid reading?

I was able to get my brothers and sisters to read the assignment. If I could hear it, I was all right, but then the next problem was taking it back and putting it down on paper again. If I did it by talking in class, I did real well, but if I had to take it and put it down on paper for a test, I got frustrated because I couldn't put down what I wanted to say.

When you were young, did you ever pick up a book and read it for enjoyment?

No. I can tell you books that were read to me, like Charlotte's Web, but for me to read a book? I bet I never . . . the only reading I ever did even until I graduated from high school was stuff I was told I had to read. It was misery. I didn't enjoy doing it, so why do it?

The thing is, with a long word, I could start it, but by the time I got to the end of it, I forgot about the beginning of the word. I'd spend 30 seconds on one word, and I'd get frustrated so I'd just skip over it. Then, I'd read the rest of the sentence and then I'd realize it didn't make sense to me. I found myself going back and starting over again. I'd start over because I was working so hard and having trouble with it, I'd forget what it was all about. I'd find myself starting all over again and not getting anywhere. That's just it. You keep on losing it because you've concentrated so hard on that one word that it's energy draining. It was such a drudgery.

CHAPTER 7

TEACHING HANDWRITING

Some students with dyslexia learn to write easily. Others, however, also have dysgraphia, a condition that makes the kinesthetic task of handwriting very difficult. Theses students have a hard time remembering what the letters look like, and they also forget how to form them. They hold their pencils tightly in an uncomfortable way and produce letters and words that do not have good spatial relationships with one another. Their writing can be very slow and labored. The main feeling about the written product is discomfort, both for the writer and for the reader, who has difficulty deciphering the text.

Why teach handwriting to such a student? Why not just teach him to type? Even with the advent of computers, people in our society are still expected to be able to write. Teachers often ask for written answers on tests. There are banking forms and job applications, and expectations from individuals, such as when one friend asks another, "Please write me a note about it." It is embarrassing not to be able to write clear, legible text. When a student can produce only scratchy, messy papers, he can be reluctant for his teachers, as well as his peers and parents, to see his work. Often, such a student becomes resistant to doing written work and will develop either withdrawal or aggressive avoidance behaviors.

Students can be taught. It requires patience and effort and structured work, but students can learn to produce legible, often excellent handwriting with comfort and ease. Even older students with bad writing habits can, with hard work, show dramatic improvement. They then have the ability to write in addition to being able to use the keyboard (which is also highly recommended and will be discussed at the end of this chapter). Most important, they can feel proud of producing legible and clear text.

SHOULD CURSIVE OR MANUSCRIPT BE TAUGHT?

It is generally accepted that all students with dyslexia should be taught cursive writing. There is some disagreement as to when this should occur. Some clinicians say that even very young students should start with cursive, whereas others argue that manuscript should be taught first and that cursive should be introduced only by late second or third grade. The latter feel that cursive letters confuse young children because they are different from the letters they see in printed text. The former assert that there is no real evidence of such confusion and that the following benefits of cursive far outweigh any possible disadvantages:

- Because students with dyslexia often have visual-motor issues with two-dimensional space, they don't know where to start a letter. Cursive writing corrects this problem, because you always start on the line.
- In print text, there are spaces between letters and between words. All those spaces and where they go can create great confusion. Cursive writing is easier because all the letters in words are connected, with spaces only between words.
- In cursive, it's natural to move the pencil from the left to the right. This, therefore, helps students with spatial issues keep their place on the page. It also reinforces the left to right movement for the tasks of both writing and reading.
- Cursive letters can be taught in groups of similar letters. With careful instruction, therefore, students can use their logical thinking skills to help them remember how to form each letter.

In this chapter, we will focus on the teaching of cursive writing.

THE FIRST STEP: BODY POSTURE

Students are often active, and they can have a habit of moving around a lot, even in their seats. A favorite posture can be a half-slouch under the table. The first thing to do is to discuss the importance of body posture with your student. Give an example, for instance, of how carpenters need to be very careful positioning their bodies when they are using tools such as saws and hammers. Pencils are tools, also, and require the same attention.

The correct body posture starts with a good chair and a table that is an appropriate height for easy writing. Because students are of different sizes, you must pay attention to the height of the writing surface. Students should be able to work with their elbows bent and their forearms approximately parallel to the floor. Both feet should be placed firmly on the floor in front of them. For a right-handed student, the paper should be placed at approximately a 45-degree angle to the left so that the corner of the paper is facing the student. A left-handed student should have the paper placed 45 degrees to the right.

THE SECOND STEP: PENCIL GRIP

The issue of how students hold the pencil can be a major barrier to instruction. An older student, especially, can have an entrenched habit of poor pencil grip and be highly resistive to change. He probably knows that he cannot write easily, but he feels that even his limited ability is dependent on that improper grip. He may be afraid that if he changes, he will never be able to write at all.

Discuss the need to hold the pencil properly with your student. Show him how to hold it between his thumb and forefinger, with his middle finger serving as a rest. Tell him that you understand how difficult it is to change, and that it *will* seem harder in the beginning as he develops his new grip. It *will* slow him down for a while. Tell him that you hope he will eventually find the new pencil grip more comfortable, and that he will able to write much more easily and quickly.

Office supply stores and some educational supply companies sell plastic pieces that fit over pencils and help assure proper grip. These can be very helpful, especially in breaking bad habits. They really help students who have been gripping the pencil so tightly that they have marks or even calluses on their fingers. After a trial period, allow your students to choose whether they wish to use these devices.

WHEN IS A STUDENT READY TO BEGIN WRITING?

When a student can stay seated in a chair and has a sense of proper pencil grip, it is time to begin practicing moving the pencil tip along the paper. Some people recommend the use of prewriting activities. For young children, they suggest forming letters out of materials such as clay or pie dough, and having the children trace their fingers along the shapes. For older students, specific exercises with the pencil are recommended, such as drawing a series of horizontal spirals. Many of these exercises can be found in the book *Cursive Writing Skills* by Diana Hanbury King (Educators Publishing Service, 1987). Activities of this type reinforce good pencil grip, help students gain muscle control, and can help students relax around picking up a pencil.

If a student is still experiencing severe difficulties with prewriting activities in spite of many attempts to help him, he may need some fine-motor exercises specifically designed for him. In this case, refer your student for an occupational therapy evaluation. If your school district does not employ an occupational therapist, consult with your school psychologist regarding how to meet you student's need and, also, to assess whether outside evaluation should be pursued.

THE INSTRUCTION TECHNIQUE

Following are the three basic principles:

1. Use large muscles to inform small ones.
2. Place letters into groups with similar beginning strokes for learning.
3. Use spoken language to reinforce the memory of letter formation.

START WITH THE LARGE MUSCLES

To begin instruction, start working with the large arm muscles. Surprise your students by telling them you are going to work on handwriting, but that you are not going to use pencil and paper. This helps in three ways. First, for the older students, especially, it distinguishes your work with them from other failure experiences they may have had with handwriting instruction in the past. Second, using the large muscles actually does help the small muscles develop motor memories of how to form the letters. It helps students experience the changes in directions that occur during cursive writing. Third, you can introduce the language you are going to connect with each letter before a student has a pencil in his hand.

A favorite technique, which has enjoyed an excellent reputation, is called skywriting. Here, you stand and model forming a letter while you simply state how you are making it. What you say has been predetermined by you and will be repeated by students when they skywrite. The letters are huge, at least three feet tall. After you have demonstrated a letter, the student then stands and copies you. Once he has done this several times and feels comfortable with the letter, he "writes" it in giant size either on a chalkboard or on large pieces of paper. For a more dramatic multisensory experience, he can "write" it in a basin of water or in a pan of sand. At this stage, help students decide which hand they feel most comfortable using to write, if they do not already have a strong preference. Let them experiment with both, and then make a choice.

PLACE LETTERS IN GROUPS

Most programs that teach handwriting to students with dyslexia place the letters in four different groups, or families. The letters are grouped according to the upstroke required to begin the letter, and emphasis is placed on always beginning the letter on the line. In most programs, the groups are approximately the same, with some slight variations. *Beginning Connected, Cursive Handwriting—The Johnson Handwriting Program* by Warren T. Johnson and Mary R. Johnson (Educators Publishing Service, 1961, 1963, 1971, 1972, 1976)—is a good example. The name of its four families and the letter groupings are

- The swing-up family with the letters, i, j, p, r, s, t, u, w
- The loop family with the letters b, e, f, h, k, l
- The up-over family with the letters m, n, v, x, y, z
- The around-up family with the letters a, c, d, g, q, o

USE SPOKEN LANGUAGE

It is very important to decide upon very simple and specific language that will become associated with the formation of the letters. This multisensory cue reminds students to slow down and concentrate. The verbalization also helps them remember the proper upstrokes and follow through.

You can choose your own words to use. For example, for the letter, "i," you can say:

Start on the line.

Swing up.

Come back down.

Release.

Dot the "i."

Keep your language simple so that it will be easy for students to remember and repeat. Most important, keep your language consistent for each letter. This way, the verbal memory and the muscle memory will be able to assist each other.

All lowercase letters should be taught first. It is best to do this slowly, with much reinforcement, so that the language cues and muscle movements are firmly connected. There is no rush to get through the alphabet. It is more effective to go a little too slowly than to rush and create confusion. You want your students to use their senses of pattern and logic, so that they perceive an individual letter as a part of a cohesive whole. When your student is asked to write a letter, you want him to think, "Oh, that's one of those in that group that starts with a tall loop. That one's easy."

OTHER CONSIDERATIONS FOR HANDWRITING INSTRUCTION

Give many opportunities for practice. The type and amount of practice will depend on the age and needs of an individual student. The first stage is to trace, which can be done on many different tactile surfaces; the second is to copy; and the third is to write the letter from memory.

If possible, practice daily. The frequency ensures a regular reminder. This is often most effective when it is done at the beginning of the day, or whenever students tend to have the most energy for learning. Concerning the length of handwriting lessons, it is most effective to have relatively short work sessions. Keeping the sessions short keeps frustration at a minimum. It is hard work for people with dyslexia to work on handwriting. They have to think about what they are doing and, on a physical level, their muscles can ache because of practicing new movements. They will try their best if they know that the session time is reasonable.

Pay attention to the size of the paper your student is using. If he is having trouble forming the letters, the paper may be too small. Provide larger pieces of paper with wider line spacing.

When using regular size, wide-lined writing paper, ask students to skip lines for handwriting practice.

Left-handed students tend to have a natural back slant. This is acceptable, and it is highly preferable to an artificial forward slant that can create a hooking of the wrist. This is a very uncomfortable and fatiguing wrist position.

When all lowercase letters are mastered, begin to teach capital letters. Teachers differ in their presentations of these. Some try to group them in terms of similar shapes. Others group them according to the beginning stroke, such as "I" and "J." In general, more variation is allowed with capitals than with lowercase letters. One handy tip is to have a sheet of paper with models for the capitals that students can keep in their notebooks and refer to readily. With practice, they will learn them.

In general, most people agree that students should begin connecting the lowercase letters once a few have been presented. Often, students practice with two letters at first and then add more. An important point is to remind students to go back to the starting line after each letter in a word. This helps them get a good start. The only letters after which this does not occur are "b," "o," "v," and "w." In these special cases, you can provide models for your student in which these letters occur. He can first trace and then copy them for practice.

As students progress with their handwriting, they are sometimes asked to copy sections of text for handwriting practice. Students with dyslexia tend to have difficulties with copying. They often will omit letters or words, or will put incorrect letters into words. This is not because of laziness or lack of effort. They simply have a great deal of difficulty with copying, often making as many errors (or more) every time they are asked to repeat a given copying task. For this reason, this type of practice is not recommended.

BE AWARE OF THE EMOTIONAL FEEL OF THE LESSON

A very important thing to remember regarding handwriting instruction is the emotional aspect of it. Many students have tried very hard to write in the past and have experienced only failure. In some ways, a person's handwriting reflects something about him, and he may have sensed unspoken criticism about not only his work but also his entire self. Some teachers and other adults who are not familiar with handwriting issues often perceive students who have trouble in this area as lazy, and unfortunately, this may have been communicated. Your student may have been forced to complete page after page of rote copying of letters, which was ineffective but certainly tiring and discouraging.

These negative experiences can make students less than enthusiastic about the idea of starting again. In the beginning, you have to believe for them that they will be able to write beautifully. Talk with them about the issues, saying things like "I know this may be hard for you, but I have a way to teach you that really is different from what has happened before. I'd appreciate it if you just tried this new approach."

One helpful thing to do is to play a trash basket-basketball game with cursive writing papers. Work for ten minutes or so on some letters, and then hold up the trash basket. Students crumple their papers and try to make a basket. They enjoy this, and it helps them relax about the cursive practice. They know that they don't have to worry about the paper forever following them, reminding them that they have difficulty in this area. It helps them be more willing to take a risk

PUBLISHED PROGRAMS

There are some very effective published programs for teaching handwriting to dyslexic students. The aforementioned *Johnson Handwriting Program*, with the booklet *Beginning Connected, Cursive Handwriting* by Warren T. Johnson and Mary R. Johnson (Educators Publishing Service, Inc., 1961, 1963, 1971, 1972, and 1976) is appropriate for younger children, because there are cartoonlike graphics. It gives a good introduction to the letters and provides pages for children to practice them.

The PAF Handwriting Program by Phyllis Bertin and Eileen Perlman (Educators Publishing Service, Inc., 1997, 1995) provides a concise teacher manual and student workbooks for both right-handed and left-handed students. An advantage of these books is that letter size is taken into consideration, and students are given opportunities first to write large, and then to decrease their letter size. The workbooks are also appropriate for any age, as there are no graphics.

Cursive Writing Skills by Diana Hanbury King (Educators Publishing Service, 1987) divides the letters of the alphabet into only two groups, those letters like "t," which begin with an upstroke, and those letters like "m," which begin with a push over stroke. The workbook provides space for prewriting exercises, practice with individual letters, and practice with words. This program is appropriate for the older student.

The *Multisensory Teaching Approach (MTA) Handwriting Program* by Margaret Taylor Smith (Educators Publishing Service, Inc., 1987, 1988) is a particularly effective program for teaching cursive handwriting to students with dyslexia. This is because it utilizes large muscles to inform smaller ones and also uses language cues to help develop memory for letter formation. You can purchase a *Handwriting Practice Guide*, which provides all the needed directions for how to teach this program, and a *Handwriting Masters* book, which gives masters that can be copied for work with students. A page from the *MTA Handwriting Program* showing the lowercase letter groupings with beginning strokes is reproduced on page 106. A page from the *MTA Handwriting Program* showing capital letter formation is reproduced on page 107.

This handwriting program is very comprehensive, and it takes some work for a teacher to learn it. However, it is also very effective.

PART 2—LETTER SHAPES

LOWERCASE BASIC LETTER STROKES

Approach Strokes

Every lowercase cursive letter begins on the baseline. Beginning every lowercase letter on the baseline eliminates the need for the writer to make decisions about where a letter begins. Placement of a baseline arrow on the writing material provides students with the place to begin, and indicates which direction to go in forming the letter. Only four basic approach strokes are used for the 26 lowercase letters. The letters are grouped according to approach strokes below.

1. Swing up, stop

→ →i →p →s →r →j →w →u

Swing up, stop

→ →t

2. Push up, over

→ →m →n →y →v →x →z

3. Under, over, stop

→ →a →d →c →g →q

Under, over, stop at the top

→o

4. Curve way up, loop left, pull straight down

→ →l →f →h →k →b

Curve up, loop left, pull straight down

→e

---

*From *MTA's Handwriting Practice Guide* by Margaret Smith (Educator's Publishing Services, Inc., 1987). Used by permission.

Capital Letters

All capital letters are three spaces above the baseline; Y, Z, and J extend two spaces below the baseline. The letters are grouped according to similar beginning strokes. It is recommended that capital letters be taught after all 26 lowercase letter shapes are mastered.

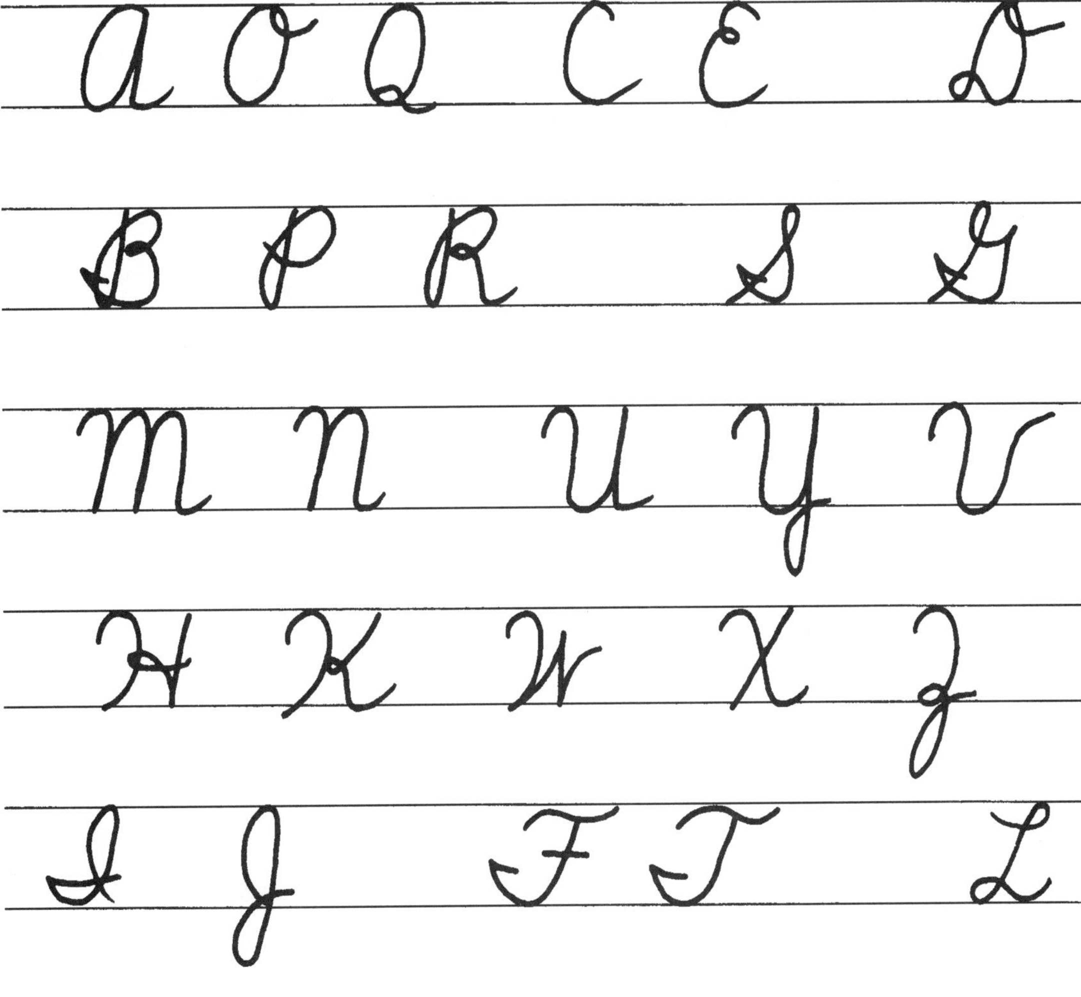

*From *MTA's Handwriting Practice Guide* by Margaret Smith (Educator's Publishing Services, Inc., 1987). Used by permission.

KEYBOARDING SKILLS

Teaching keyboarding skills as soon as your students are ready is an excellent idea. Often, they tell you this by their willingness to practice. The program that is highly recommended is *Keyboarding Skills* by Diana Hanbury King (Educators Publishing Service, 1988). The premise of this program is that students should use the alphabet, an already meaningful language tool, to learn the keyboard. Thus, students are taught proper posture on the keyboard, and the placement of fingers on home keys. The first letter presented is "a," and then "b," and so on. Students practice by typing rows of these letters and then combining them into alphabets. Once they know all the letters, they begin typing first two-letter words, and then three-letter words, and so on. This very effective technique really works for students with dyslexia.

INTERVIEW WITH JEREMIAH

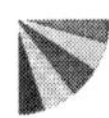

Jeremiah is a 15-year-old boy who attends a public high school. He is very talented in art and in mathematics. He faces challenges with dysgraphia, dyslexia, and ADD. Jeremiah has never received remediation for his issues with handwriting.

Let's talk about handwriting.

My mom was talking a while ago how when she saw me in third grade, she saw me do chicken scratch handwriting, holding tight onto the pencil and shaking, and then two minutes later, I'd be sitting there drawing delicate things. And she was amazed that the same hand could in five minutes do something completely different.

And it's weird, because it's completely brain related. I like switch over, and when I switch over, it's like a burden is completely off my back. I don't have to have trouble handwriting any more. I can now draw a face or something.

Why do you think you draw so beautifully and have trouble with the handwriting? How does it feel to you inside?

It feels, it's like, let's say that you're great at making a soufflé, but you're horrible at making chocolate mousse, and you don't know why. You're making all these kinds of foods, but this one kind of food, every time you make it, it burns. Every time you do it, something happens and it turns out wrong and horrible. It's the same way with me. I can draw perfectly, I mean not perfectly, but very well, and then I turn around and do writing; I can't make my letters look good unless I spend five minutes drawing the letters.

It's like, if I make it creative, I can write, but if I have to do a form, kind of, I have trouble with that. I don't know why it happens. It's just that it reaches a certain point, and then it's a different part of the brain.

Has it always been that you've had trouble with handwriting, ever since you were a little kid?

You know how when you're a little kid, you have those lines where you have to make a big "A" and then a little "a." One page you do an "s," and the next page you do "b." I had problems with those. I've had problems, ever since those. My handwriting got worse, because I realized I can just scratch. I don't have to take fifteen minutes to make letters, so it makes the writing more enjoyable, even though I'm the only one who can read it.

Actually, it's kind of legible, but it makes it more enjoyable because I don't have to worry about my handwriting. I can just say, "I know what this means." So I can then type it on the computer or read it to somebody who can then type it. So, that's been helpful. My handwriting has always been—if I spend a lot of time on it—it can look semidecent, but if I don't, my normal handwriting is pretty scratchy.

So, motor output issues affect your handwriting and keyboarding?

My hand gets tired doing stuff like that. When I'm drawing, it's weird, I don't know how to compare—it's like I get a time-out when I'm drawing. I can draw for hours, and it won't hurt my hand. But, like, I took a couple of hours of notes the other day and I got calluses on my hands because when I'm writing, I have to hold my pencil as hard as I can, and then I still kind of make messy letters and I get kind of confused and flustered, and it's really annoying.

And typing—it's weird because if I'm playing on the computer, it's no problem to do all those things, and then I go out and type and I don't want to type. My hand doesn't want to.

"Is that because language is involved?

It's like my brain has trained itself to not like writing. It's more of a subliminal thing than it's a decision of mine that I'm not going to enjoy writing. In fact, I like making up stories and being creative, but then I don't want to get those out, which is really why I like this View Voice. Then I can make up long stories. (View Voice is a program that enables the computer to type out the spoken word.)

What's so hard about handwriting?

One hypothesis I have is that it's the same every time I do it. There's no element of change. Every time I make an "r" it has to look like an "r." I can't change it. I can't make my "r" backward. It has to be the same so that people will understand it.

But with my drawing, it has to look different every time. If you draw the same thing again and again, people will say, "Oh, this is boring." I like things that you can change. I like being able to say, "Oh, this picture, I don't like this eye and I'm going to change it."

If I don't like my "r," I can't erase it and make it different. "R" is kind of like a universal language. I mean, with a painting, everyone can tell that it's a cat or everyone can tell that's a flower, because if you had the leaf different, you could still tell it was a flower. And like a face, it doesn't have to look like anybody in the entire world, I can freeze it. Everybody knows it's a face.

But if I make an " r" backward, the loop at the top and the line at the bottom, no one will know what that is. It doesn't exist—it's theoretical. That's why I don't like doing the same letters. I'm bored with them, I'm tired of doing them over and over. If you eat the same cereal every day, you get sick of it. I'm sick of the same letters; I want different letters. I'd like to make up a different set of letters and make everybody in the world learn them.

But the problem is that I have a hard enough time with these letters. That is my hypothesis up to now. It's like a subliminal thing. I'm not sitting here saying I want to change the letters, It's like I have this little part of me sitting on my shoulder saying, "I want new letters, it's boring, change the letters." But then the other part of me says, "No, if you want to fit into society, you have to learn them."

CHAPTER 8

TEACHING SPELLING

Most students with dyslexia experience difficulty with spelling. This is especially true because of the way spelling is taught in our schools today. The typical instructional method is for the teacher to present a number of words on Monday, then ask students to practice with these words during the week and supposedly master them by Friday. The better programs attempt to present words that share some predictable patterns, but even these programs usually intersperse irregular words and many phonetic variations. Students are basically expected to memorize the series of letters that make up the words.

This approach does not work for students who have difficulty with memory, especially the rote memory of relatively meaningless strings of letters. Some teachers have tried to create lists of words that are meaningful for the student with dyslexia. They have taken words from the student's writing and high-interest words that occur in content areas that are being studied. This is a serious attempt to help the student with dyslexia. It also is not effective, because the words themselves may be meaningful but their spellings aren't.

What, then, works? Students with dyslexia are generally very smart and intellectually curious, and they have good logical thinking skills. They are able to see and utilize patterns. These strengths can be used to teach them to spell. They usually do not become terrific spellers, and they don't sign up for spelling bees. They can, however, learn to spell very adequately. They can learn to spell well enough to effectively use computer spell checks, and even though spelling is usually not a strength for them, they can learn to feel comfortable and capable with it.

HOW TO TEACH SPELLING—THE BASIC APPROACH

The tremendous contributions of Dr. Samuel Orton and Anna Gillingham to the teaching of the language skills of reading and spelling were discussed earlier in this resource. One of the unique aspects of their approach is to teach the structure of the

English language. Even though many English words have been borrowed from different languages and this gives great diversity to the spelling, it is estimated that English is approximately 85 percent phonetically regular. Once a student understands the structure of this majority of the language, she can use her logical thinking skills to predict spelling patterns. She then has to develop compensatory strategies for only the other 15 percent.

Whole-language philosophy also informs our work with spelling. It shows us that if students feel some connection with the words being studied, they will approach spelling instruction in a more motivated and relaxed way. This will aid memory. Even though students with dyslexia generally have *poor* memory skills, that does not mean that they have *no* memory skills. They *can* learn to memorize many high utility irregular words, especially if they are not being asked to memorize hundreds of them.

The recommended approach, therefore, is an integration of phonetic strategies with whole-language philosophy. It is taken from *Spelling Smart! A Ready-to-Use Activities Program for Students with Spelling Difficulties* by Cynthia M. Stowe (The Center for Applied Research in Education, 1996). This book contains detailed information on the techniques and issues summarized below. It also presents complete instructions for teaching 40 lessons.

THE FIRST STEP: THE ALPHABET

ASSESSMENT

As with reading, it is important to assess your student's knowledge of the connections between letters and sounds. Don't assume with an older student that she knows all her sounds. She may not, and work at this level may have to be done before formal spelling instruction can begin.

First, see if your student knows all her consonant sounds. Give her a lined piece of paper and say, "Please number your paper from 1 to 24, skipping lines." Wait, and then start the exercise with the instructions given at the top of the sheet on page 115, "Diagnostic Screening for Consonant Sounds."

If your student knows most of her consonant sounds, next assess her ability to hear and record the short vowel sounds. These sounds are particularly difficult for the student with dyslexia. Give her a lined piece of paper and ask her to number it from 1 to 25, skipping lines. Then, begin this exercise with the instructions given at the top of page 116, "Diagnostic Screening for Short Vowel Sounds."

Assess not only your student's knowledge but also her comfort level with the task. This gives important information about her degree of confidence.

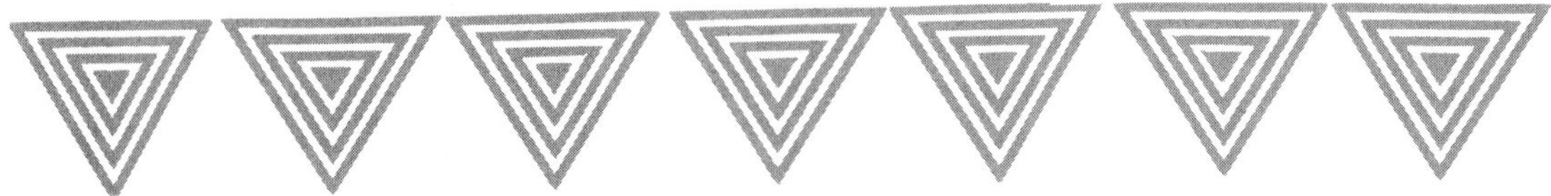

Diagnostic Screening for Consonant Sounds

For Spelling

Provide a lined piece of paper and say, "Please number your paper from 1 to 24, skipping lines." Then say, "I am going to say some sounds. When you hear the sound, please write down the letter that represents that sound. Most of the time, I will not give you a word associated with the sound. I will do that only when more than one letter represents a given sound."

SOUND	CORRECT ANSWER
1. /d/	d
2. /m/	m
3. /k/ as in "cat"	c
4. /t/	t
5. /s/ as in "sit"	s
6. /l/	l
7. /g/ as in "game"	g
8. /w/	w
9. /h/	h
10. /j/ as in "jam"	j
11. /b/	b
12. /kw/	q
13. /f/	f
14. /z/ as in "zipper"	z
15. /r/	r
16. /j/ as in "giant"	g
17. /ks/	x
18. /n/	n
19. /s/ as in "city"	c
20. /y/	y
21. /k/ as in "kite"	k
22. /v/	v
23. /z/ as in "is"	s
24. /p/	p

Diagnostic Screening for Short Vowel Sounds

For Spelling

Provide your student with a pencil and lined paper. Ask her to number her paper from 1 to 25.

Say, "The first thing that I'm going to ask you to do is to write the five vowels on your paper from 1 to 5. Sometimes, the letter 'y' is used as a vowel, but don't put that one down. List the other five vowels."

When your student is finished, say, "I am now going to say some words that begin with a short vowel sound. After I say the word, write down the vowel it begins with. If you're not sure, take a guess." Dictate numbers 6 to 15.

WORDS	ANSWER
6. Odd	o
7. Act	a
8. End	e
9. It	i
10. Us	u
11. Enter	e
12. Opposite	o
13. Imperfect	i
14. Adolescent	a
15. Uncover	u

Say, "I am now going to say some words that have vowel sounds in the middle of the word. Listen carefully, and then write down the vowel you hear in each word." Dictate numbers 16 to 25.

16. Cup	u
17. Tap	a
18. Pit	i
19. Bell	e
20. Sod	o
21. List	i
22. Pond	o
23. Rust	u
24. Bent	e
25. Camp	a

If your student shows a lack of knowledge of letter sounds, it's important to do some work in this area. General principles of teaching letter-sound connections are:

- Use multisensory instruction. Have students see, hear, and say the information.
- Connect the sound with a key word.
- Teach one sound at a time until students are comfortable with them.
- Provide frequent chances for practice and review.
- Make sure that you are presenting single sounds, as opposed to blends. In other words, teach "b" says /b/ as in "bat," as opposed to "br" says /br/ as in "bread."

To illustrate the basic technique of teaching a letter sound for spelling, let's look at how to teach the consonant sound "t." Gather together some objects and some pictures of objects that begin with the letter "t." Discuss these with your students.

Next, say the following words, " tap," "top," "time," "team," "toe." Ask your student, "What sound do you hear in the beginning of these words?" When she is able to tell you that she hears the /t/ sound, write the five words on a piece of paper or on the chalkboard. Say, "What do you see at the beginning of all of these words? When she can tell you that she sees a "t," proceed to finding a key word for the letter.

Key words are important because they help create a memory of the letter sound connection. Decide on a key word that is meaningful to your student, and write that word on one side of an index card. Write the letter that the key word represents on the other side. If the key word for the letter "t," for example is "table," have your student practice with the cards in this way: "'T' says /t/ as in 'table.'" At every lesson, have your student practice with her deck of index cards, which will grow as more and more letters are learned.

Short vowels are taught in essentially the same way. For students with dyslexia, short vowels can be very difficult to discriminate between and to remember. For this reason, teach the short vowels, but do not expect your student to have mastery of them before you start spelling instruction. The spelling program itself will reinforce the learning of these sounds.

Occasionally, you'll have a student who has severe difficulty with discriminating between letter sounds, blending sounds, knowing how many sounds are in a word, and knowing the order of these sounds. For these students, the *Lindamood Phoneme Sequencing Program* is recommended. Extensive training is required to teach this program. Consult with an appropriate professional, once you have obtained permission from the student's parent or guardian, and describe the needs of your student. Further diagnostic work may need to be done to see if this program is appropriate for your student. For more information on the *Lindamood Phoneme Sequencing Program*, see pages 70 and 71 of this resource.

An effective spelling program for students who have difficulty seeing in their minds the spelling of words is *Seeing Stars, Symbol Imagery for Phonemic Awareness, Sight Words and Spelling* by Nanci Bell (Gander Publishing, 1997). This program focuses on helping students learn to visualize the spelling of words. It is a highly structured program that needs to be taught with care. Once done so, however, it can be very effective.

BECOMING FAMILIAR WITH THE STRUCTURE OF THE ENGLISH LANGUAGE

Most of us were never given information about the structure of the language. To feel comfortable with using the approach recommended here, therefore, it is helpful to first learn a little about it:

- There are 21 consonants. These letters represent units of sound which usually end quickly, like the sounds of "p" and "t." Consonants such as "m" and "l" can be continued with the voice, but a part of the mouth or the lips are generally closed.
- Certain combinations of consonants can have unique sounds, such as "sh," which represents /sh/; "ch," which represents /ch/; "ph," which represents /f/; and "th," which represents /th/.
- There are six vowels: "a," "i," "o," "u," "e," and sometimes "y." These letters represent sounds that can go on indefinitely, limited only by the amount of breath a person has. The mouth is usually open. Vowels can be pronounced long, for example, when "i" says its name as in "hi." Vowels can also be short, for example, when "i" says /i/ as in "him." The vowel "y" can say long /e/ as in "penny," or short /i/ as in "gym."
- Several combinations of vowels represent unique sounds; for example, "oo" represents the /oo/ sound, as in "moon."
- Several combinations of consonants and vowels represent unique sounds, as when "ble," represents the /bul/ sound in "table."
- Words are composed of units of sounds called syllables. Syllables each have at least one vowel, and varying combinations of other letters. For spelling, we present six types of syllables in the English language:

  1. *Closed syllable:* A single vowel is stopped or closed in by a consonant, as in "it" and "cat."
  2. *Vowel-consonant-e:* A vowel is followed by one consonant, which is immediately followed by an "e." In this type of syllable, the vowel is long, as in "pine."
  3. *Open syllable:* A single vowel is not followed by a consonant, and thus, the mouth could conceivably stay open. Two examples of open syllables are "go" and "me."

4. *Vowel combination syllable"* Two vowels combine to make one sound, as when "ai" says long /a/ as in "rain."

5. *Consonant-le syllable:* This type of syllable occurs only in a multisyllabic word. It is made up of a consonant like "p" or "d," combined with "le." Words like "maple" and "handle" are the results.

6. *R-controlled syllable:* The letter "r" exerts its powerful influence on any vowel that it follows. For example, the "a" is neither short nor long when it is followed by an "r," as in "car."

- Specific rules help us know how to correctly add endings to base words. Following are the three main rules in the English language.

1. *The "E" rule.* When a suffix that begins with a vowel is added to a word that ends in "e," the "e" is dropped, as in "bake" + "ing" = "baking." When a suffix that begins with a consonant is added to a word that ends in "e," the "e" remains, as in "plate" + "ful" = "plateful."

2. *The doubling rule.* When a suffix that begins with a vowel is added to a one syllable word that ends in one consonant, preceded by one vowel, the last letter of the word is doubled, as in "run" + "ing" = "running." When a suffix that begins with a consonant is added, no doubling occurs, as in "sad" + "ness" = "sadness."

3. *The "Y" rule.* When a suffix is added to a word that ends with "y," the "y" changes to an "i" if the "y" is preceded by a consonant, as in "happy" + "ness" = "happiness." If the "y" is preceded by a vowel, the "y" remains, as in "stay" + "ing" = "staying."

- There are also some spelling generalizations. Two important ones are:

1. *The "ff," "ll," "ss" spelling generalization.* In a one syllable word that has a single short vowel and that ends with "f," "l," or "s," you double the last letter, as in "puff," "hill," and "pass."

2. *The "ck" spelling generalization.* The /k/ sound is spelled with "ck" when it comes directly after a short vowel at the end of a word, as in "check."

THE SECTIONS OF THE LESSON PLAN

Once your student has learned most of her consonant sounds, and is at least familiar and somewhat comfortable with the short vowel sounds, it is time to begin formal instruction. The parts of the lesson plan are very structured and predictable for students. This helps them relax, because they know what is going to happen and they also know that they will be asked to do only what they are able to do. They will not be expected to copy long lists of words or to memorize spellings. They will be successful from the first time they pick up their pencils and make a mark on the paper.

There is no set amount of time for each lesson. Begin with a section, work at your student's pace, and proceed to the next section when it seems appropriate. You can spend as little as fifteen minutes on a part of a lesson, or as much as an hour.

A positive approach is critically important as work is begun. Your student will probably not feel confident initially, so you must feel confident for her. Tell your student something like this: "I understand that you have had difficulty with spelling in the past. In the past, you were asked to memorize words, and that was difficult for you. Some people have good memories for spelling and other people do not. Not being good at this doesn't have anything to do with intelligence. Very smart people can have trouble memorizing spelling.

I am going to show you a new way to learn spelling. You will learn about how the English language has evolved and about the structure of it. You will learn predictable patterns in the language, which you will be able to use to spell. In time, spelling is going to become much easier for you."

The sections of the lesson plan follow.

GETTING STARTED

This is a very important part of the lesson, because here students review previous information. Often, they use their spelling notebooks during this time. It is recommended that every student be given a looseleaf three-ring binder into which she can place information that she has written about the language. She can also keep prior lessons in this notebook, as well as other important information.

INTRODUCING NEW INFORMATION

Here, you create situations in which students discover spelling patterns. They thus become active participants in their own learning. You don't *tell* them; rather, you help them *discover* information in two ways. First, you help them to hear a sound that is being presented. Next, you help them to see the letter that it represents.

For example, to teach the short vowel sound for "a," you can do the following:

Say the following words: *am, bat, fan, band, map, rag*.

Say, "What sound do you hear in all of these words?

That's correct, /a/ as in ant. It's called short 'a.'"

Write the following words: *am, bat, fan, band, map, rag*.

Say, "What letter do you notice in all of these words?

That's right, the letter 'a.' Today, we will be studying words that have short 'a' in them."

Practicing with Individual Words

Dictate 8 to 15 words to your students, which she will write down with a pencil with a good eraser. It is recommended that she write on wide-lined, not college-lined, paper. All of the words in the word list presented will contain two things:

1. The phonetic element that is being studied
2. Only phonetic elements that have already been presented, with which you know your student is at least relatively comfortable

The first assures that your student will be able to practice with the new information that she has just discovered. The second gives her the opportunity to practice with any elements that she has previously studied. It also assures success. She will be able to spell all the words presented. She may have to think about it and to concentrate, but she will be able to do it independently.

Once students have written down their words, it is time to help them self-edit their spelling. This is critically important, because most people who have had problems with spelling in the past have experienced an excessive amount of teacher correction. They get back their papers all marked up in red. They often feel frustrated and overwhelmed, and a common reaction is to give up. Why focus on something that seems so impossible? Also, even if all this teacher correction has been done in a nurturing way, it still reinforces the idea that *someone else* is responsible for their spelling.

To help the student begin to notice her own spelling and to take responsibility for it, first ask her if there are any words in her list of which she is unsure. If there are, and if a word has been spelled incorrectly, guide your student back to the relevant information that has been presented with careful questions. For example, pretend that you have been studying the spelling generalization that for single-syllable words with one vowel that end with the letters "f," "l," or "s," you double the last letter, as in "stuff," "hill," and "class." Your student has spelled the word "smell" in this way: "smel."

Show your student the list of words that you originally presented to introduce this spelling generalization. Ask her, "Look at how you've spelled "smell." Do you think that's right?" Let her correct her own work.

Once your student has asked all her questions, ask to see her work. If she has incorrectly spelled any word, ask her leading questions so she will notice the error.

Your main goal is to help your student begin to notice her own spelling and to begin to take responsibility for it. Once she does, she will be emotionally able to focus much more of her energy on her work.

Practicing Spelling in Context

In this part of the lesson, approximately four sentences are dictated. These sentences have been carefully prepared to contain only phonetic elements that have already been presented. If there are phonetically irregular words, which are sometimes necessary to include, especially in the beginning of instruction when not many elements have been introduced, students should be given a model for each irregular word. Write each one on a separate piece of paper and place them in front of your student.

First, show your student the sentences that she will be writing. Ask her to look them over and see if there is anything that confuses her. Answer questions and talk about any unusual vocabulary. Then, dictate each sentence completely. If your student asks you to repeat it, read it through completely again. This is a good technique for improving auditory memory, and it also reinforces the concept that words occur in context.

When your student has finished writing all her sentences, ask her if there are any words that she is unsure about. Readily give her the spellings for any words she requests. This is different from the procedure with individual words, in which you respond only with a guiding question, because people who have had difficulty with spelling often are overwhelmed by writing sentences. It helps them risk more to know that they can simply ask you how to spell any word they wish once they are finished.

At some point, when your students are more advanced and have become quite confident, you may return to answering their questions with a guided question of your own, as you do with individual words. Use your instincts as to when this becomes appropriate.

Once your student has completed her questioning, ask her if you may see her work. If there are any errors, place one small check mark in pencil for each error on the side of the line. Then, deal with one error at a time. Point to a check mark and say, "Can you find the word in this line that needs to be changed?" Once she has found it, help her to correct it with guided questioning. As soon as it is corrected, erase the pencil mark. It is important that when your student completes her lesson, she has produced as neat a paper as she can. There are no red correction marks anywhere.

REINFORCING ACTIVITIES

Whole-language philosophy has influenced this section of the lesson. Here, students either recognize or utilize the phonetic elements they have been studying. Even though this part of the lesson tends to be less structured, it is very important. Here is where information can be fully internalized.

These activities can also help with the pacing of lessons. It is hard work for a student with dyslexia to work on spelling, and she needs to move slowly and carefully so that she doesn't get overwhelmed. Generally, it's better to err on the side of going too slowly rather than introducing material too quickly. Once your student has mastered the elements presented, she will want to move forward.

Reinforcing activities can be quite diverse. The following are some examples (phrased as if you are speaking to your students):

1. (This activity is offered once short "a" and short "i" have been introduced.) Make phrases with words with short "a" and short "i" in them; for example, "the slim man," "a frantic kid," and "a fantastic rabbit." Write sentences using these phrases or draw illustrations for them.

2. (This activity is presented once short "o" has been introduced.) Play a game with a friend or two. Write down ten closed syllable words with short "o" in them where everyone can see them, like "cot," "mop," and "hog." The first player mentally selects a word and then writes it down secretly on a piece of paper. The other players ask questions to which there is a "yes" or "no" answer. For example, "Does your word represent an animal?" A total of ten questions may be asked. The first person to guess the word gains a point, and he selects the next secret word. If no one guesses the word after ten questions, the first player gains a point and selects another word.

3. (This activity is appropriate at any time.) Play Concentration with a friend. Take index cards and write the words you are studying, one to a card. Make two cards of each word. When you have made approximately ten pairs of words, place them face down on the table. The first player turns two cards over. If they match, she keeps them and she has another turn. If not, she places them face down again, and the second player gets a turn. The winner is the person who collects the most cards.

4. (This activity is presented once words such as "time," "dime," "mice," and "pine," have been studied.) Have you ever heard the cliché "Time will tell?" It means that, in time, the answer to many things will become obvious. Think for a moment, however, about the specific words used in this cliché and about their literal meaning. Then, illustrate this literal meaning. For example, you could draw a picture of a clock that is talking. If you wish, also illustrate the cliché "He can stop on a dime."

5. (This activity is presented once words such as "cure," "flute," and "huge," have been introduced. It is a Literature Connection activity appropriate for students in grade 5 and up.) When Chinese people first came to America, they brought with them a rich folklore. "The Cure" is one such story. It can be found in the book *Tongues of Jade* by Laurence Yep (Harper Collins, Publishers, 1991). In this book, Mr. Yep has translated and retold many Chinese-American tales. "The Cure" is a story of magic. Another story in *Tongues of Jade*, however, deals more directly with issues of human nature. Read "The Teacher's Underwear" and enjoy a humorous and poignant tale.

Extra Interesting Facts

In this last section of the lesson, you can offer some interesting piece of information about the history of the English language, or something fascinating about the origin of a specific word. To find such information, you can refer to books such as *The Story of English*, a companion to the PBS television series by Robert McCrum, William Cran, and Robert MacNeil (Viking Penguin, 1993). You can also check the stories of individual words in etymology books. A favorite is *Word Origins and Their Romantic Stories* by Wilfred Funk (Random House, 1992).

The purpose of this section is to interest students in the history and evolution of the English language. This curiosity often helps them have more patience with the vagaries of English spelling.

A SAMPLE LESSON

The following lesson is taken from *Spelling Smart! A Ready-to-Use Activities Program for Students with Spelling Difficulties* by Cynthia M. Stowe (The Center for Applied Research in Education, 1996). This sample lesson illustrates all of the lesson sections listed above. It also provides activity sheets for this sample lesson. They are the following:

- ***Finish It!:*** Students select words from a word list to complete sentences.
- ***A Game of Categories:*** Students select words from a word list and place them in one of four categories.
- ***Look It Up!:*** Students look up ten presented words and then use these words in sentences.
- ***List It!:*** Students write a list that deals with the sameness of all people.
- ***Write On!:*** Students write a short piece of prose about their opinions of smoking cigarettes.

  These same types of independent activity sheets can be prepared for all the different lessons. They are provided in *Spelling Smart!*

  At the end of this chapter, five more independent activity sheets are offered. All of these activity sheets may be reproduced and used for any spelling pattern you wish. They are:

- ***Word Teams:*** Students select pairs of words and then use them in sentences.
- ***Write It Again . . . and Again . . . and Again:*** Students select individual words and then use each one as many times as they can in a sentence.
- ***Use Them All:*** Students select some words and use as many as they can in a paragraph.
- ***Magic Box Word Game:*** Students fill a prepared grid with letters and then try to make words.
- ***Spelling Bingo:*** Students fill in an empty grid with words they are studying and then play Bingo.

SAMPLE LESSON
THE E RULE

Getting Started

Ask your students to look through their notebooks and to tell you anything they wish about the structure of the English language. Discuss what they introduce.

Ask your students to tell you what they remember about the suffix "ed." Provide time for your students to make a notebook page for this suffix.

Introducing New Information

"Today, you are going to discover your first spelling rule."

Write the following words on the board or on a large piece of paper: *bake, drive, hope, make, smile, tune*.

"What type of syllable do you see in all of these words?"

"Yes, they all contain vowel-consonant-e syllables. What letter do they all end in?"

"It's obvious—they all end with the letter 'e.'"

Write the following formulas:

chase + ed = chased
vote + ing = voting
brave + est = bravest

"What happened when you added a suffix to these vowel-consonant-e words?"

"That's right, the 'e' was dropped and the suffix was added."

Write the following formulas:

home + less = homeless
like + ness = likeness
plate + ful = plateful

"What happened when you added a suffix to these vowel-consonant-e words?"

"I agree; nothing happened. The 'e' was not dropped and the suffix was added."

Place the two sets of formulas in front of your students and ask, "Can you figure out why, in some cases, the 'e' was dropped, and in other cases it was not?"

"That is correct. When a suffix that begins with a vowel is added to a word ending in 'e,' the 'e' is dropped. When a suffix that begins with a consonant is added to a word ending in 'e,' the 'e' remains."

Practicing with Individual Words

Select a manageable number of words from the word list provided on page 128 for your students to spell.

Practicing Spelling in Context

Select a manageable number of sentences from the following list for your students to write:

Ben is driving home to Memphis.

"This film is exciting," Pam said.

The graceful actress waved to them.

The convict escaped and ran up the hillside.

Meg and Beth hiked and then camped next to the lake.

Bob hoped that Jane had saved the sick rabbit.

"It is shameful that that man is homeless," Jim said.

As she smiled, Fran said, "Mike is joking."

Dave disliked the man, and accused him of making a rude statement to the press.

"It is not taking Steve much time to run that six miles," Bruce said.

Reinforcing Activities

Allow your students to choose from the following list of activities:

1. Select pairs of words, one in which the "e" is dropped when a suffix is added, and one in which the "e" remains; for example, "saved" and "graceful," and "hoping" and "lateness." Make sentences with these words. An example for the last pair is, "She was hoping that her lateness would not be a problem." If you wish, illustrate one or more of your sentences.
2. Play charades. Make a pack of at least ten cards, each of which has either an action word or a phrase written on it. Some examples are: "skating," "escaping," "riding a bike," "driving a bus," or "baking a cake." Then, get some friends together and divide them into two groups. One player selects one card and acts out the word or phrase for her group to guess. If the group guesses successfully within a given time period, they get a point, and the other group tries its luck with a new card. The group with the most points at the end wins the game.
3. The cliché "all fired up" means that a person is full of enthusiasm and excitement. As you can tell, however, the literal meaning of this phrase is quite different. Illustrate the literal meaning of "all fired up."

4. LITERATURE CONNECTION: Sometimes, the bravest people among us start out afraid. This is the case with Albert Brooks, the hero in *The Contender* by Robert Lipsyte (Harper Collins, 1967). Albert has dropped out of high school and is struggling with fear—fear of the bullies around him, fear of his own lack of opportunity in life.

Albert takes positive action, however. He joins a gym and begins to train to be a boxer. Read *The Contender* and discover how Albert becomes one of the bravest people on his block.

Extra Interesting Facts

Some of our English words come from two words being pushed together; for example, the word "smog" comes from the combination of "smoke" and "fog." In this case, not only the "e" was dropped but also the "k," along with the "f" in "fog."

Other English words are the result of two words being connected; for example, "baseball," "bareback," "driveway," and "fireplace." In these cases, no letters are dropped. It's interesting to think about how both old words contribute to the meaning of the new word.

There is one main exception to the "e" rule you have discovered in this lesson. When a word ends with a soft "c" or a soft "g," usually the "e" is kept, even if the suffix begins with a vowel. Examples of such words are "traceable" and "manageable."

WORD LIST

One-syllable words:
The "e" is dropped.

(as in bake + "ed" = baked)

baked	probed
bravest	riding
chased	ripest
dining	saved
driving	shaking
faded	shining
framed	smiled
hated	taking
hiked	traded
hoped	voted
joking	waved
making	widest
named	

One-syllable words:
The "e" remains:

(as in ape +"s" = apes)

apes	mutness
blameless	pavement
cuteness	plateful
graceful	rudeness
grateful	rules
homeless	shameful
hopeful	spiteful
hopeless	statement
hugeness	themes
jokes	timeless
lateness	tireless
likeness	wakeful
miles	

Multisyllable words:
The "e" is dropped.

(as in accuse + "ing" = accusing)

accusing	exciting
admired	exploded
dictated	invading
disliked	invited
engaged	inviting
escaped	misplaced
escaping	stampeded
excited	

Multisyllable words:
The "e" remains.

(as in athlete + "s" = athletes)

athletes	hillsides
bagpipes	hotcakes
basement	placement
confinement	potholes
cupcakes	trombones
engagement	vapires
flagpoles	wishbones
gemstones	

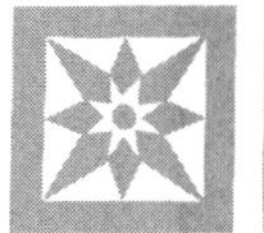 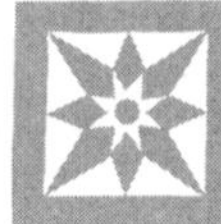  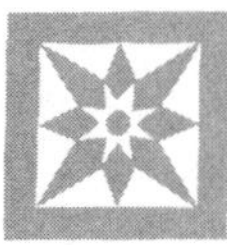  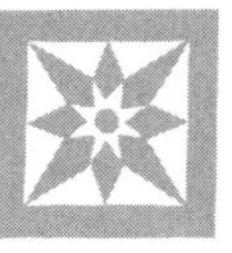 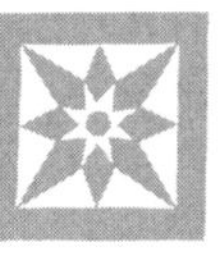 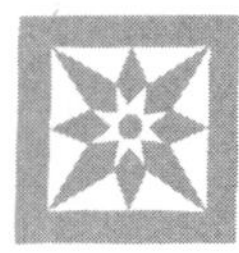 

FINISH IT!

Fill in the blanks with words from the word list.

1. The little girl _______________ her friend around the schoolyard.
2. The townspeople _______________ the mayor for his honesty and courage.
3. "I am still _______________ that I will be able to come to the party," Helen said.
4. On election day, Fred left home early and _______________ before he went to work.
5. Ben _______________ his best hat and could not find it.
6. "You are _______________ if you wear your seat belt," Mike said.
7. Peg has been _______________ horses in shows since she's been eight years old.
8. At the Halloween costume party, there were several _____________ .
9. On Saturday, Tom _______________ ten loaves of bread.
10. They went to the _______________ room for supper.

WORD LIST

hopeful	voted
misplaced	riding
vampires	baked
admired	chased
dining	safest

Name ________________________________ **Date** ________________

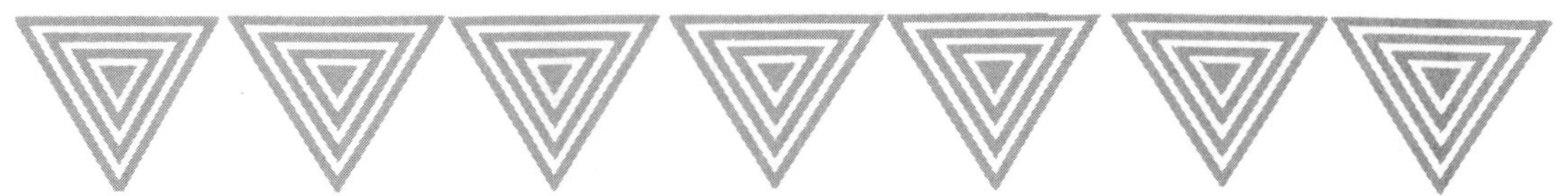

A Game of Categories

Choose words from your word list that belong in each category.

RELATING TO FIRE AND HEAT	RELATING TO MOVEMENT
____________	____________
____________	____________
____________	____________
____________	____________
____________	____________

RELATING TO HAPPY FEELINGS	WORDS THAT DESCRIBE FOOD
____________	____________
____________	____________
____________	____________
____________	____________

WORD LIST

fires	ripest
admired	smoked
flames	hiked
hoping	boneless
riding	baked
stalest	excited
blazing	biked
smiled	glazed
sliding	driving

Name ______________________ **Date** ______________

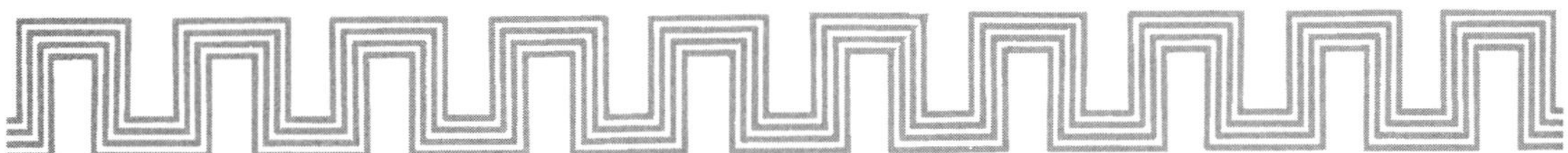

Look It Up!

Look up the listed words in your dictionary. Then match each word with its correct definition.

1. anecdotes	a. referred to
2. pruning	b. gave out a certain portion
3. crazed	c. appearing to cut short, or be cut short
4. meted	d. trimming a plant
5. glazed	e. wanting success or what success can buy
6. alluded	f. putting into bondage
7. enslavement	g. covered a surface with a smooth finish
8. imbibing	h. little stories, often of a personal nature
9. truncated	i. drinking
10. aspiring	j. frantic

Please choose five words from this list and use each one of them in a sentence.

1. ____

____

2. ____

____

3. ____

____

4. ____

____

5. ____

____

Name ____________________ **Date** ____________

List It!

People are all different, but our sameness is more compelling than our differences. Make a list that deals with the sameness of all people. For example:

1. We all need air to breathe.
2. We experience feelings such as joy or anger.
3. All people must be cared for when they are born.

See how many ways you can think of that illustrate the sameness of all people.

____

____

____

____

____

____

____

____

____

____

____

Name ______________________ **Date** ______________

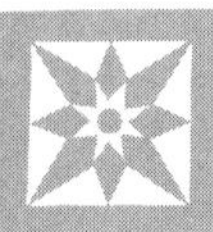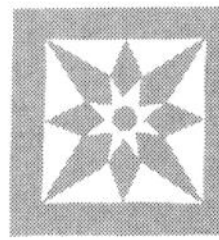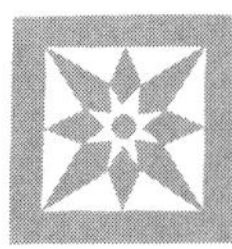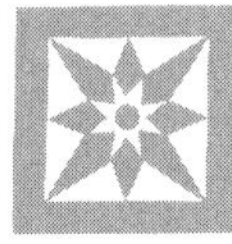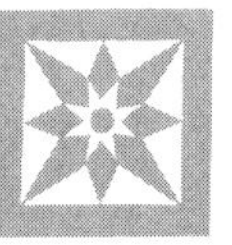

Write On!

Smoking Is Hazardous to Your Health!

Have you ever seen or heard that slogan? What do you think about smoking cigarettes? Do you feel that it is fair for a business to restrict the right of people to smoke in its space? Do you feel that nonsmokers have more rights than smokers because of the danger of breathing in secondhand smoke?

Write your opinion about smoking here. You can discuss one of the questions mentioned above, or you can write about a different issue that relates to smoking.

____

____

____

____

____

____

____

____

____

____

____

Name ______________________________ **Date** ________________

ANSWER KEY FOR SAMPLE LESSON WORK SHEETS

Finish It!

1. chased 2. admired 3. hopeful 4. voted 5. misplaced 6. safest 7. riding 8. vampires 9. baked 10. dining

A Game of Categories

RELATING TO FIRE AND HEAT: fires, flames, blazing, smoked, baked

RELATING TO MOVEMENT: riding, sliding, hiked, biked, driving

RELATING TO HAPPY FEELINGS: admired, hoping, smiled, excited

WORDS THAT DESCRIBE FOOD: stalest, ripest, boneless, glazed

Look It Up!

1. h 2. d 3. j 4. b 5. g 6. a

7. f 8. i 9. c 10. e

RECOMMENDED SEQUENCE FOR INTRODUCING PHONETIC ELEMENTS

Introduce short vowels first. Even though these are often difficult for students with dyslexia to hear and to discriminate between, it's important to work with them in the beginning of a spelling program, because then students can use them and practice with them as they proceed. Because there are so many words in English that have short vowels, this makes it possible for you to create interesting sentences for your students to write in the "Practicing Spelling in Context" section of the lesson.

One caution: Don't expect mastery of the short vowels before you move on to the next phonetic element in the sequence. As long as your students have some sense of the short vowels and can successfully spell words with them most of the time, it is best to move on. They will continually practice with them in their dictated sentences.

The following is the recommended sequence:

1. Closed-syllable words with the short vowels "a," "i," "o," "u," and "e"
2. Vowel-consonant-e syllable words with "a-e," "i-e," "o-e," "u-e," and "e-e"
3. Open syllable words with "a," "i," "o," "u," and "e"
4. Vowel combination syllables "ai," "ay," "ee," "oa," "ea," "oo," and "ow"
5. Consonant-le syllables "ble," "dle," "ple," "gle," "tle," "fle," "cle," and "kle"
6. R-controlled syllables "ar," "or," "er," "ir," and "ur"

The spelling generalizations, such as how to use "ck" at the end of a word, and the three main spelling rules, the "e" rule, the doubling rule, and the "y" rule are presented interspersed throughout the sequence.

OTHER IMPORTANT ISSUES RELATED TO SPELLING

IRREGULAR WORDS

Because the portion of the language that is phonetically regular is focused upon, not much attention will be placed on these words. There are a few common irregular words, however, that are convenient for students to be able to write; for example, "the," "said," "of," and "to." There are different ways to make these words accessible to students.

- Provide a written model when the word is needed.
- Make a card deck of ten or so very common irregular words that the student can refer to whenever she desires.
- Have students record very common irregular words (not more than twenty or it becomes cumbersome) in their spelling notebooks for future reference.

For more advanced students, you may wish to occasionally take a break from the standard spelling curriculum and complete an actual lesson on irregular words. Two types of words are recommended for this work:

1. A group of words that have something in common, even though they are irregular
2. High-visibility words that your student may want to know

An example of the first type is words with silent letters, such as "knot," "sign," and "write." An effective way to help students remember these spellings is to tell them that it is believed that, in the past, these silent letters were pronounced. Students can enjoy pronouncing the words in the old fashioned way.

An example of the second type is the names of the days of the week or months of the year. Make a list of the words you are working with, and notice any words that follow phonetic patterns that have already been studied. Then, for the truly irregular ones, use etymology to make the spellings interesting, as opposed to merely torturous.

HOMONYMS

Homonyms are words that sound alike but that have different meanings and spellings. They are extremely difficult for students with dyslexia. They should be introduced only as a supplement to the regular program once students have become comfortable with closed syllable, vowel-consonant-e, and open-syllable words. It's helpful to use etymology and to present these homonym teams as interesting aspects of the English language.

The following is a sample lesson for teaching the homonym team "there," "their," and "they're."

1. Introduce the following chart for students to complete. Challenge them to find the word that doesn't need the capital.

Word	Sentence to be completed
Their	__________ is a strong wind blowing.
They're	The students got into __________ car.
There	__________ going to go to the basketball game.

Ask your students to figure out which words belong where. Tell them they can consult with other people if they wish.

2. Provide as many sentences as are needed for your students to gain a sense of the meaning of each word.
3. Once the meanings are clear, record each word with its meaning and a sample sentence on cards or on a chart that is highly visible to students.
4. Ask your students to record this information in their notebooks.
5. Allow your students to use these models for as long as they wish to do so. They can be expected to edit their own work for the proper spelling of the homonyms.

COMPUTER SPELL CHECKS

Computers and spell check programs are wonderful inventions that can greatly help the student with dyslexia become independent with spelling. If spell checks are to be used effectively, however, students must first gain a certain level of spelling competence. If they have not, the computer will not recognize the word that is desired, or it will highlight or underline so many words in a text that it is extremely discouraging for the writer. Computers also do not yet discriminate between homonyms. Thus, students should be encouraged to use spell checks only when they are already competent spellers.

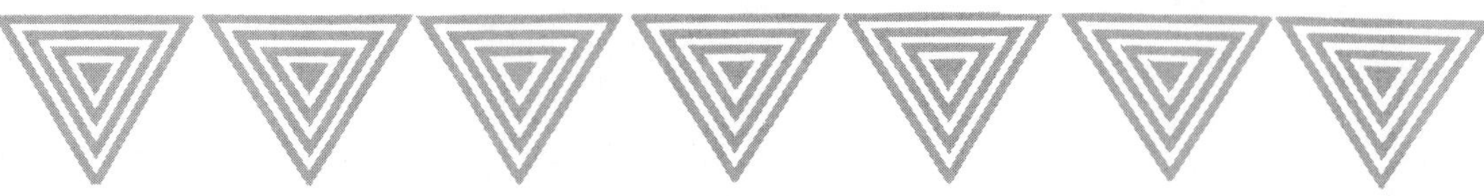

WORD TEAMS

Choose pairs of words you have been studying. Then, use these pairs in sentences. For example, if your pair is "grass" and "glass," you could write, "There was some broken green glass in the grass."

________________ ________________

____

____

________________ ________________

____

____

________________ ________________

____

____

________________ ________________

____

____

________________ ________________

____

____

Name ______________________________ **Date** _________________

WRITE IT AGAIN . . . AND AGAIN . . . AND AGAIN

Choose a word with a pattern in it that you have been learning to spell. Then, see how many times you can use that word in a sentence. For example, if your word is "train," you could write:

"The train was fast, because the train had been made in a train factory that made fast trains."

Can you beat this record of using a word four times? Good luck!

____

____

____

____

____

____

____

____

____

____

____

____

Name ______________________ Date ______________

USE THEM ALL

Choose five words from a pattern you have been studying. Then, see if you can put them all in one good paragraph. For example, if you select the words: "drove," "phone," "hole," "home," and "smoke," you could write:

When Kim drove to her friend's home, she saw an amazing thing. She saw smoke coming from a hole in the road. Kim avoided the hole and went on. As soon as she got to her friend's house, she used her phone and called the fire department. "I'm not kidding," she said. "You've got to investigate that smoke coming up from the road."

_______________ _______________

_______________ _______________

____

____

____

____

____

____

____

____

____

Name ______________________ Date _______________

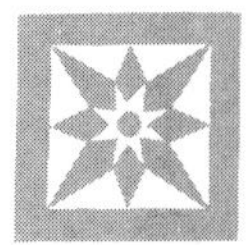

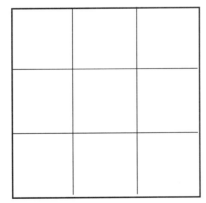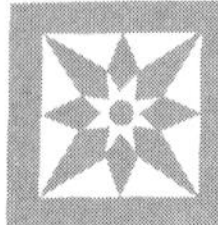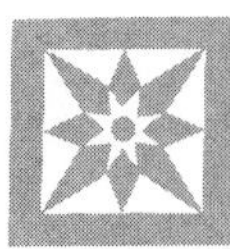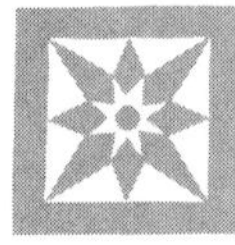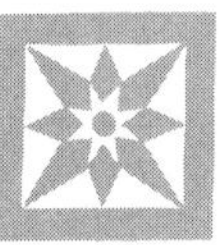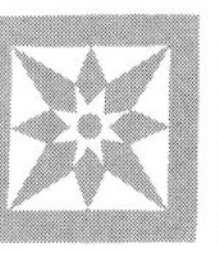

MAGIC BOX WORD GAME

Make as many words as you can by combining the letters in the box below. Each letter must touch the one before it.

c	m	r
n	a	t
f	s	b

Words: (for example: cab, rat)

____

____

Now, fill in letters to make your own magic box game.

Words: ____

____

Name ______________________ **Date** ______________

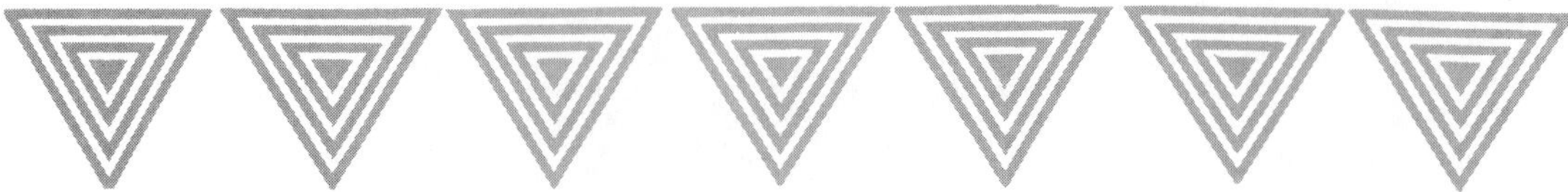

Spelling Bingo

Select fifteen words that have a spelling pattern you have been studying. Then, make a card pack by writing each of these words several times on index cards.

Next, fill in each square below with one of your words. You can repeat words in any way you wish.

To play "bingo," the caller mixes the cards and then reads them from the top. If one of your words is called, color in one of your squares with that word in it. The first player to complete either a horizontal or vertical row wins the game.

Name ______________________ **Date** ______________

Interview with Jeremiah

Jeremiah, who spoke in Chapter 7 about dysgraphia, tells about the challenges he faces with spelling.

Let's talk about spelling

Spelling has improved a lot. I used to not be able to spell anything. I used to spell cat with a "k." Like, my name I couldn't spell. I mean, it took me a while to spell my name. My name's a hard one, so that's why I like to be called Jeremy, because Jeremy is pretty simple. We shortened it, so I could remember how to spell that. It's like six letters. Jeremiah is eight letters. It's harder, plus it's got all those "ia"-"ai" things where you're not sure how they go, and I got all flustered with my name. But now, I know that really easily.

This is the worst language I could have been born in, in which there are too many rules and everything's not spelled right. Spanish is hard for me because I had a hard time with English, and now I have to learn Spanish, too? That's just stupid, I shouldn't have to be doing that, I should be working on English.

But Spanish is easier. Spanish is like, it's always spelled this way and there are two rules—this or this. I'm like, "Okay, I can speak the language." I mean, I can't really speak the language. I mean, it took me 15 years to remember all the words in English, and now, I'm going to remember all of them in Spanish in 6 months? But I wish I had started in Spanish.

I don't wish that I'd started in Spanish, because this is my favorite country in the world, and I love America. America's cool, and I like English because English is probably the most spoken language in the world. Because, in America, you speak English. In Japan, you speak Japanese and English, and in Spain, you speak Spanish and English, and in Russia, you speak Russian and English.

I wish English was easier. I wish that the base language was easier. English is one of the hardest languages, so I go for one of the hardest languages, and then I have trouble with it.

So spelling, it's kind of, it's sort of, it's difficult because there's too much to remember. I can't memorize all the words. I try to remember the important ones, and then I stumble over the harder ones. I've gotten better at remembering the rules. I used to try to memorize every word. I'd go over it and over it, and say, "All right, I've got this word."

Now, what I try to do is kind of, like in math, I get the formula down. I plug in my x and y values, and out comes the answer. I get my answer by plugging in the different variables I have. So, like with the word "Atlantic," I say, "Okay, there's an "At" and a "lan" and a "tic." And most of the time it works. Some time it fails, and that's when I use spell check, or Mom or my sister says that's wrong. So I'm getting to the point where I know enough rules and I've had enough experience spelling that I'm okay.

In fourth grade, I was so discouraged. I felt like, "I can't spell. I don't know how to spell. I'll never be able to spell." I used to do horrible in my spelling tests, but now I realize that, in fourth grade, I'd only learned it for three years, and now I've learned it for another six. Now, I have nine years of experience instead of three. It's getting easier.

CHAPTER 9

TEACHING WRITING

Students with dyslexia often are reluctant writers. This is *not* because they don't have a lot to say or that they are not talented in this area. In fact, once students receive appropriate instruction, they often show that they have unusual talent. They display original, unique, and effective ways of expressing their thoughts and feelings. But think for a minute about what the task of writing involves. You have to be able to form letters (or type) easily, to spell effortlessly so that it doesn't slow down your thought processes, and to use English grammar rather automatically. Then, you can focus on presenting and organizing what you want to say. Finally, it's important to be able to read what you have written. Is it any wonder that students with dyslexia do not automatically enjoy writing? What person would, given the difficulties of the tasks listed above? With proper instruction, however, students with dyslexia often become excellent writers. And, equally important, they can learn to enjoy the work.

THE PROCESS OF WRITING

The process of writing—in other words, how to begin putting that first word or sentence on the paper and how to organize effectively as you continue—must be taught. It is also recommended that reading and writing instruction be integrated for optimal effectiveness. Because all of the aforementioned skills of cursive writing, spelling, and knowledge of grammar are so intertwined with writing, it's important to be aware of all of them as you proceed.

The following approach is taken from *Let's Write! A Ready-to-Use Activities Program for Learners with Special Needs* by Cynthia M. Stowe (The Center for Applied Research in Education, 1997). Basic tenets of this program are the following:

1. There is sequential presentation of the skills needed for successful writing. Students begin by writing words, then sentences and paragraphs, and then finally stories, essays, and reports. Students are successful from the very beginning.

2. The experiential approach is used. Instruction is provided in a way that allows students to be active rather than passive learners. This helps them be more motivated and to have fun as they work.

3. Multimodality instruction is provided. Students' areas of strength are recognized and utilized, and they immediately begin to realize that they can become good writers.

4. Students are expected and allowed to be independent from the very beginning of the program. Activities are structured so that students can always do the writing themselves. This helps build self-esteem and gives them important practice at the level at which they are working.

5. Structures for written language are provided. For example, it's taught that a paragraph begins with a topic sentence, has supporting detail sentences, and finishes with an ending sentence. Although these structures are not always rigidly adhered to, they give a logical way for students to begin organizing groups of sentences. Students with dyslexia appreciate and understand structure. Why not use this strength in their writing?

6. Each lesson consists of four different parts that utilize different skills. This diversity within the lesson helps active students stay focused on their work. As an example, one lesson of moderate difficulty could include the following:
   - Write a list of things that you can put on your hands.
   - Write a paragraph about why rain forests are important (after there has been reading about rain forests and discussions about the topic).
   - Play a game that involves pantomiming verbs.
   - Listen to a teacher read aloud a section of a book, such as *Letters from Rifka* by Karen Hesse (Henry Holt, 1995).

7. Many interesting and different opportunities for writing are provided. Students improve as they practice writing. The challenge is to help them enjoy doing so.

THE BASIC SEQUENCE FOR INSTRUCTION

Start at the beginning for all students and make sure that they are competent with basic skills. Many students with dyslexia spend much of their available energy compensating and, yes, even hiding their weaknesses, especially when they first start working with you. Therefore, it's best to check the basics. The worst that will happen is that you will spend a little extra time finding out that your student has some good basic competencies. And he will have a successful experience showing you what he knows.

The following teaching sequence is recommended:

1. Word Writing
2. Sentence Writing
3. Paragraph Writing
4. Writing Research Reports, Book Reports, and Stories
5. Writing Essays

How to teach each of these is discussed below.

Word Writing

Students need to be aware of sound-symbol correspondence as they begin this work. If they have not yet mastered all the connections between sounds and letters, instruction should be provided in a separate part of the day. Information on how to do this is provided in Chapter 6 of this resource. Separate instruction in both areas of sound-symbol correspondence and word writing can be mutually supportive.

Many beginning writers are reluctant and, at times, openly resistive to the task. Usually, this is because they have experienced a great deal of failure in the past. Just holding a pencil has been problematic, and spelling isn't so easy, either. Why should they want to display their difficulties in black and white?

You can begin by talking with these students. Tell them that you understand that they don't really like to write. Writing has probably been hard for them in the past, and people don't usually like to do what is difficult. You are going to teach them in a different way, however, and this will make writing easier for them.

The critical element is success. Students have to be successful from the first time they pick up their pencils. It is critical to structure lessons so that this can happen. The two basic principles of teaching word writing are:

1. *Provide as much modeling with oral and written language as your students need.* Some students will have difficulty with thinking of a word that they wish to write. You can give them the word; for example, if they are looking at a picture of a tree but can't seem to say anything, you can say, "I notice that you are looking at that picture of a tree." If your student is just beginning with written sound-symbol correspondence, provide written models for the words he wishes to write. This does not inhibit him from writing on his own. On the contrary, students usually start writing independently when they are ready.

2. *Present lessons that are as concrete as they need to be so that your students are successful.* For example, at the most basic level, provide concrete objects. You can either bring in interesting objects or gather some from the room. Place them on the table and say, "Let's write down what's here. Ah, we have a shell and a marble and a top." Students seem to enjoy this activity even if it is repeated many times. Change the objects, and get your students writing those words.

The following three activities are excellent for the development of word writing skills:

1. **Write lists of words.** These lists can be of objects on the table. Other ideas are: things in the room, things that can be put into a sandwich, colors, and jungle animals. Students can look at pictures and books to get ideas for their lists. An independent activity sheet, "A List," is provided on page 149.
2. **Do labeling.** Students either cut pictures from old magazines or draw their own. They can label individual objects or the parts of them. For example, if your student draws a car, he can label and draw arrows to the wheels, hood, steering wheel, and windows.
3. **Make and play games.** A good example is the game Concentration. Have students write about eight pairs of words, one word per index card. Place all sixteen cards face down on the table in random order. The first player selects two cards. If they match, he has another turn. If they don't match, he places the cards face down again, and the next player has a turn. Keep adding new words and eliminating old ones, and your students will get a good amount of word writing practice.
4. **Play the category game.** Provide a list of words and at least two categories. For example, you can write the two categories "Food" and "Clothing," and give models for the words "pizza," "hat," "shoes," "hot dog," shirt," and "potato." Ask your students to write the words in their appropriate categories. An example, "A Category Game," which can be used as an independent activity sheet is provided on page 150. This activity sheet is appropriate for a beginning writer. As your students advance, you can give them up to four categories.

SENTENCE WRITING

The basic principle of providing enough support for your student to be successful also operates at this level. To the student who has never before written a sentence, this task can seem daunting. Therefore, you must build a bridge, so that he will be writing complete sentences before he even realizes it. There are three levels of support.

At the first, or **basic level,** you write short sentences on the board or on a large piece of paper, such as:

- I like cats.
- I like movies.
- I like elephants.

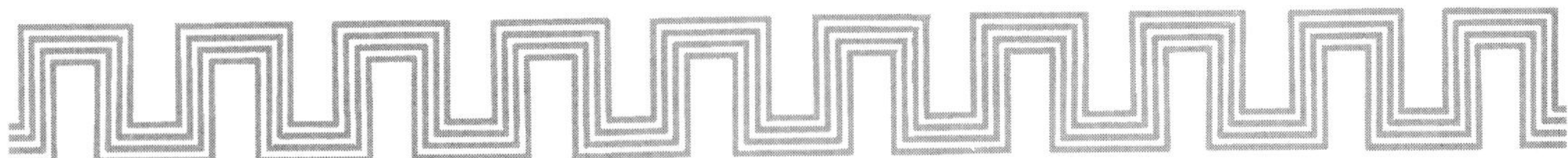

A List

Think about an apple. Then, imagine that you are holding it in your hand and looking at it. Notice how big it is. Then, make a list of things that are smaller than your apple, such as a penny or an eyelash. Look around the room for good ideas.

____

____

____

____

____

____

____

____

____

____

____

____

____

Name ______________________ **Date** ____________

A Category Game

Choose words from your word list that belong in each category.

ANIMALS	PARTS OF THE BODY
____________	____________
____________	____________
____________	____________
____________	____________
____________	____________

WORD LIST

pig	rib
rat	bat
lip	chin
hand	hen
cat	hip

Name ____________________ **Date** ____________

Tell students that you are going to give them a model for part of the sentences they will write. Then write,

- I like . . .

Ask your students to copy the model and then complete the sentence. Have them continue with this task for as many sentences as is comfortable. They are, in effect, still word writing, but they are getting the "feel" of writing sentences. Some other sentence starter models are:

- I saw a . . .
- It was fun to . . .
- Dogs are . . .

At the second, or **intermediate level**, provide sentence starters that are less important to the content of the sentence. Here, students are asked to provide their own phrases, as opposed to only words. Some good sentence starters at this level are:

- On Mondays, I . . .
- My favorite kind of TV show is . . .
- If I could fly, I would . . .

At the third level, or **more independent stage**, students are almost ready to write sentences on their own. Here, you provide just a bit of help to get them started. Some good examples of sentence starters are:

- I wish . . .
- It's not fair that . . .
- Sometimes, ...

At this level, students are often very concerned about their spelling and will ask repeatedly for the correct spelling of words. If possible, encourage them to do the best they can, but not to worry about their spelling. You want them to get used to expressing themselves freely. Tell them that, if they wish at a future time, you will help them edit their own work for correct spelling. This should be at a separate time, however, from the writing process.

Once students are able to begin writing sentences independently, provide many opportunities for them to do so. Some students prefer creative writing, while others prefer nonfiction. Allow them to work in the area in which they feel most comfortable.

It's important to spend adequate time at the sentence writing level, even for students who are somewhat capable of going on to the paragraph writing stage. Sentences are the building blocks of written language. The more competent students feel with them, the easier it will be to make the transition into longer works.

The following three activities offer practice for sentence writing skills:

1. **Write lists.** This is the same activity as with words, but the lists are different in that complete sentences are required. List topics can include "This is why I was late this morning" and "This is what I would do if I was in charge of the world." An independent activity sheet, "A List of Sentences," is provided on page 153.
2. **Conduct interviews.** Brainstorm a series of questions with your student and write them down in complete sentences on the board or on a large piece of paper. Have your student copy his favorite questions. Ask your student to interview someone, and have him either tape-record or take notes during the interview. Once the interview is completed, ask him to write out the answers in complete sentences. Then, if he wishes, he can prepare a presentation about the person he has interviewed for a small group. "An Interview," an independent activity sheet on page 154, offers examples of questions.
3. **Write "About Me" sentences.** Beginning writers often feel most able to write about themselves. Provide topics such as "Tell me about your favorite foods" and "Tell me some of the things you'd like to do when you're older."

PARAGRAPH WRITING

Beginning to write well organized, fluent paragraphs is a big challenge for the student with dyslexia. For this reason, a structured way of writing paragraphs is first introduced. Tell your students that you are going to show them how to write paragraphs that have a very specific pattern:

- One topic sentence
- Three supporting detail sentences
- One ending sentence

This pattern will help them become comfortable with writing longer, connected pieces of text. Once they have practiced enough with this particular pattern, they will be able to move on and write paragraphs that are more varied but that are still easy to read and very logically structured.

Begin this work in the following way:

1. *Discuss topics with your students.* Make a collection of topics, writing each one on a separate index card. Then, model the creation of topic sentences, such as "This is what I like about playing basketball." If you wish, you can write a topic on one side of the card, and a possible topic sentence on the other.
2. *Model the development of supporting detail sentences.* First, select a topic and create a topic sentence. Then, brainstorm for possible supporting detail sentences.

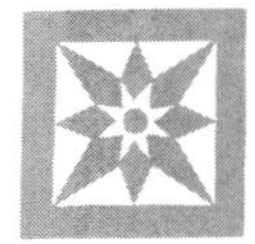 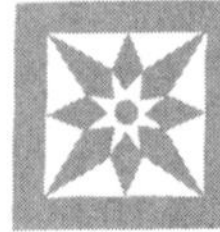 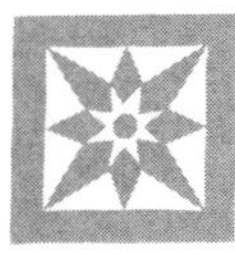  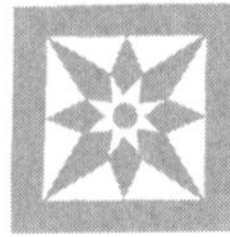  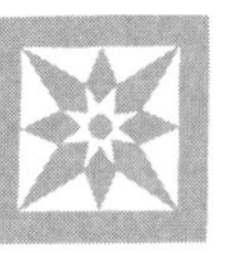 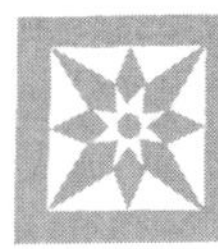 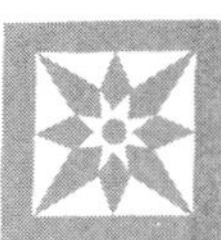

A List of Sentences

You are standing on the shore of a big lake and you want to get to the other side. Make a list of ways that you can travel across this body of water. If you want to add extra challenge, think of ways that do not involve using any kind of boat, for example:

I could catch a ride on a really big fish.

I could ice skate across, if the lake was frozen.

____

____

____

____

____

____

____

____

____

____

____

Name ________________________ **Date** ______________

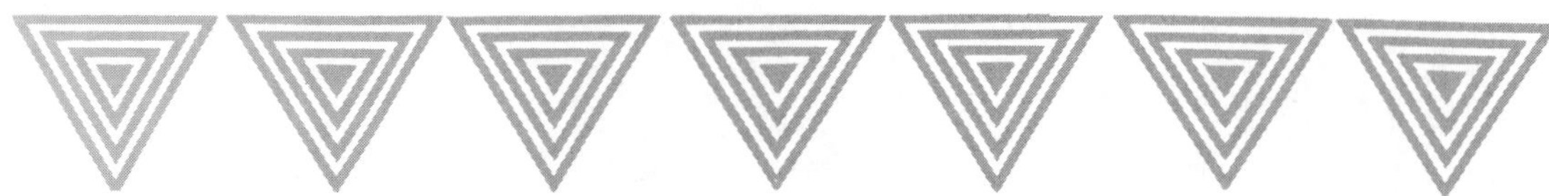

An Interview

Write the answers in the spaces provided. If the person you are interviewing does not wish to answer any question, thank the person for telling you that and skip that question.

1. What do you like to eat for breakfast? ______________________________

   ____

2. Please describe a favorite piece of clothing. ________________________

   ____

3. What is your favorite holiday, and why do you like it? _______________

   ____

4. What do you enjoy doing during your free time? ____________________

   ____

5. What is your favorite kind of work? ____________________________

   ____

6. If you could go to a special place and live there for a year, where would you go, and why? ______________________________________

7. If you could grant a special wish to a friend, what would you grant, and why? ____

8. If there were one thing you could change about the world, what would that be? ____

Name ____________________________ **Date** ________________

At this stage, it's helpful to write each sentence on a separate index card. These can be color-coded; for example, the topic sentence can be written with blue ink, and the supporting detail sentences with green. This distinguishing feature helps students internalize the different purposes of the two types of sentences. Once you have cooperatively created many supporting detail sentences, let your student write some on his own.

3. *When your student is very competent with the prior two steps, introduce the concept of the ending sentence.* Model the development of this type of sentence, as follows:

   Topic sentence

   Cities can be nice places to live.

   Three supporting detail sentences

   There are many other people around who can become friends.
   Hospitals and churches can be nearby.
   Public transportation can help you get around.

   Ending sentence

   I really enjoy living in the city.

As with the topic sentence and supporting detail sentences, you can write the ending sentence with another color of ink, perhaps red or purple, to distinguish it from the previous sentences. Some students have difficulty with the ending sentence because it seems similar to the topic sentence. Tell them that the ending sentence is a place where they can express an opinion. This often helps them begin to write this type of sentence.

A form for students to write this structured paragraph is provided on page 156. It is strongly recommended that you use this form, as its physical structure really helps students begin this type of work. When students are ready to make the transition to regular paper, have them follow the same physical pattern for awhile. Introduce standard physical structure (indenting for the beginning of a paragraph and continuing on with the other sentences) only after students are very secure with writing paragraphs in the patterned way.

Once students are clear about paragraph structure, they need to practice a lot in order to continue developing their skills. Often, teachers find this can be a problem because students have a limited range of what they feel comfortable writing about. One technique that helps is for you to read aloud a small selection of interesting nonfiction text. Then, ask students to write a paragraph about what they have just heard. An excellent source for text selections of this type is *Reading Stories for Comprehension Success: 45 High-Interest Lessons with Reproducible Selections and Questions That Make Kids Think* by Katherine L. Hall (The Center for Applied Research in Education, 1997). There are two books in this series, one for the primary grades and one for intermediate. Even though these books are intended to be used to develop reading comprehension, they can also be very useful for assisting the development of writing skills, and they can be used with all ages up to adult.

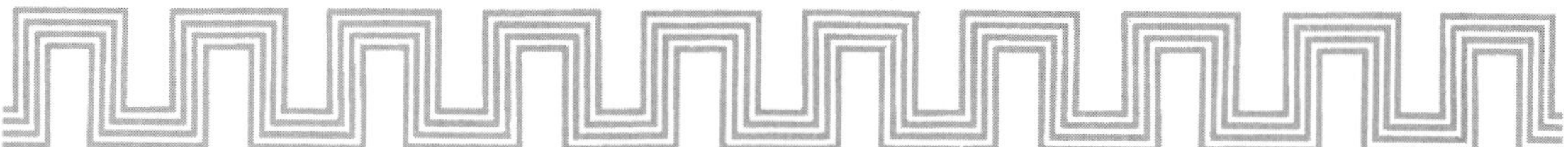

A Paragraph

TOPIC SENTENCE

____

____

THREE SUPPORTING DETAIL SENTENCES

1. ____

____

2. ____

____

3. ____

____

ENDING SENTENCE

____

____

____

____

____

Name ______________________ **Date** ______________

The following two activities can also provide practice for writing paragraphs:

1. **Write "what if" paragraphs.** Propose a "what if" possibility, and ask students to write their reactions to it. Some good ones are:

   - What if you won the lottery?
   - What if you could swim to the depths of the ocean?
   - What if you met the Loch Ness monster?

   An example of a "What If" independent activity sheet is provided on page 158.

2. **Write "Can You Beat This?" paragraphs.** Provide a topic sentence such as "My little sister is the smartest kid in the world," and let your students have fun exaggerating. Other topics are:

   - My friend Leslie has the funniest looking car in the city.
   - I ate more than anyone else for dinner.

An example of a "Can You Beat This?" independent activity sheet is provided on page 159.

Writing Research Reports, Book Reports, and Stories

The basic tools for writing are the abilities to write words, sentences and paragraphs, and most attention has been given to the direct, structured work for the development of these. The writing of research reports, book reports, and stories, however, can support the development of these basic skills. They are also important in themselves, as they are the types of writing that will be expected by teachers throughout students' school careers. Basic information on how to present these types of writing follows.

Research Reports. The most important thing to consider is the level at which students are comfortably writing: word, sentence, or paragraph. Good reports that are satisfying to both writer and reader can be written at all three levels. *At the most basic word writing level,* ask students to draw pictures and to label them. If, for example, a student is studying the civil rights movement, he can draw a map of places where important events (such as marches and speeches) occurred, and he can then label them. Another excellent report writing activity at the word writing level is list writing. If your student is studying the Civil War, for example, he can write a list of the pieces of clothing and other gear that were issued to soldiers on both sides.

At the sentence writing level, you provide a topic sentence that your student then answers with a list of sentences. For example, if he is studying the animals in Alaska, you can provide him with the following: "These are some of the animals that live in Alaska." If he needs a model to begin, write the following on a piece of paper, "The ____________ lives in Alaska." As with all sentence writing work, provide as much support as is needed.

A "What if" Paragraph

What would you do if you woke up one morning and discovered that you could fly? Would you tell anyone? Would you travel to interesting places? Write a paragraph like the one below to say what you would do.

> This is what I would do if, one morning, I discovered that I could fly. First, I'd check it out a little by flying around my room. Then, I'd clean up the mess that I made because I wasn't too good at this flying thing and so I knocked over my lamp. Then, I'd call up my best friend to tell him what was happening. Flying is a little scary, but it's also fun.

____

____

____

____

____

____

____

____

____

____

Name ______________________________ Date ____________________

     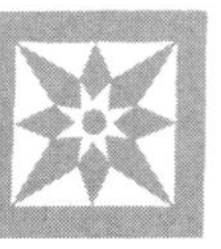   

A "Can You Beat This?" Paragraph

Write a paragraph that begins with the topic sentence, "Yesterday, I encountered a lot of wild animals." Try to exaggerate even more than in the following paragraph.

> Yesterday, I encountered a lot of wild animals. First, I found a boa constrictor in my bathtub. Then, I met a baby hippo on my back steps. When I went to school, I found a zebra in the library. There were so many animals, I could have started a zoo.

____

____

____

____

____

____

____

____

____

____

____

Name ______________________________ **Date** ________________

At the paragraph writing level, help your student develop three or more good topic sentences that he wishes to work with in his report. Provide as much support as is needed in helping him follow the structured format of the topic sentence, supporting detail sentences, and ending sentence.

For students who are ***able to write paragraphs independently***, introduce them to the following format for writing a report:

- An opening paragraph telling what the report will be like
- Several paragraphs that present information
- An ending paragraph that can form conclusions or express opinions

In effect, this structure is very similar to the original paragraph pattern, and this helps students become less intimidated by "having to write a long report." By breaking reports down into manageable sections, they can relax.

Book Reports. The first thing to consider when approaching this type of task is the prior experiences your students may have had. Sometimes, if they have experienced a great deal of failure with traditional book report writing, it is best to first focus on alternatives to the traditional form. Activities such as designing a book cover with back-cover copy, making posters advertising the book, writing book reviews, and writing invitations for a presentation and then dressing up as a character and giving a "talk," are good examples of these alternatives.

Once you feel that your student is ready to try the more traditional form, provide writing opportunities at the level at which he is comfortably writing. If he is working at the word writing level, provide questions that require one word or short-phrase answers. Do the same for working at the sentence and paragraph levels. If your student is writing paragraphs independently, provide some guidance and structure for what is usually included in a book report. Help him develop some good topic sentences. Then, give him time to work.

Stories. In many schools, writing stories is the favored form of writing instruction. Students are often given some stimulus to begin with, such as "Write a story about an animal who has a magical power." Then, they are told to work for a half hour or more, after which the class will come together and share. For the student with dyslexia, this can be extremely intimidating. Even though he may have an excellent imagination and sense of humor and could write a fabulous story if given proper guidance, the less structured nature of the instruction leaves him uncomfortable and blocked. He sits at his desk, pencil in hand, "thinking." Often, not much writing gets done.

If an older student has had many such experiences in the past, he may be reluctant to write stories. He also may have a true preference for writing nonfiction. The best thing to do for either case is to offer interesting creative writing opportunities at the level at which students are comfortable. These are some examples of story writing activities:

1. **At the word writing level, draw a picture of an exciting event.** Students first draw a picture and then label the characters and any important objects. An independent activity sheet, "Look What's Happening" is provided on page 162.

2. **At the sentence writing level, write a serial story.** Here, people write in teams of at least two. The first person writes one sentence to begin a story and then passes it on to the second person, who writes the second sentence. They continue on for as long as they are excited and interested in their story. The only two rules are that each person can write only one sentence at a time, and that no one can "kill off" another person's character. An independent activity sheet, "A Serial Story," is provided on page 163.

3. **At the paragraph writing level, write a type of story called "A Very Long Excuse."** Here, you present a topic such as "This is why I didn't do my homework" or "This is why I just had to eat your plate of spaghetti." Tell your student that after he acknowledges his transgression, he can have a lot of fun making up a story for why he did it. An independent activity sheet, "A Very Long Excuse," is offered on page 164.

The most important point with creative writing is that it has to be joyful. Present some relatively easy and enjoyable opportunities for writing, and see how engaged your students become. The main key is, if they are actively writing, allow them to continue. If they are sitting passively for long periods of time or expressing distress in other ways, invite them to do some other type of writing.

Writing Essays

This form of writing will be introduced only to your more advanced writers. It's important to work at this level, however, when students are ready to do so, because they will be expected to write essays throughout their school careers. If they can learn to begin writing easily on a variety of subjects and to clearly organize what they know about a topic, this will help them immensely.

For the student with dyslexia, starting an essay is often the hardest part. For this reason, a specific technique is recommended. First, brainstorm a series of topics with your students. These can cover the following possibilities:

- Specific topics such as racism or television programming
- Opinion statements about political issues, such as, "Is it important to vote?"
- Opinion statements about personal and moral issues, such as "What would you say to a friend who is anorexic?"

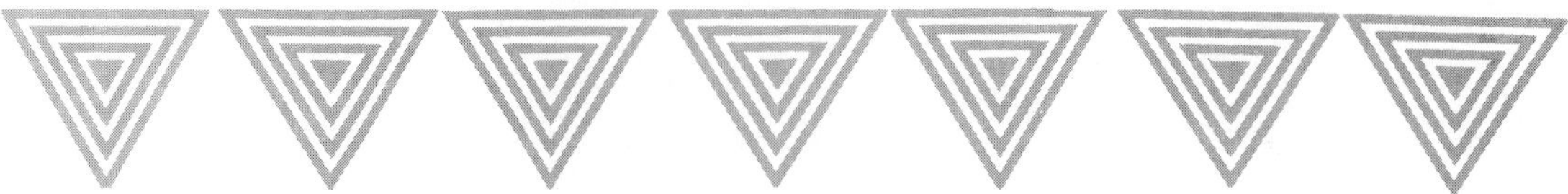

Look What's Happening

Imagine that you are walking along with a friend. All of a sudden, an armored car drives by, and a large bag falls out of the back. It looks like a bag of money!

Draw a picture of what happens. Label the main characters and any important objects.

Name ______________________________ **Date** ________________

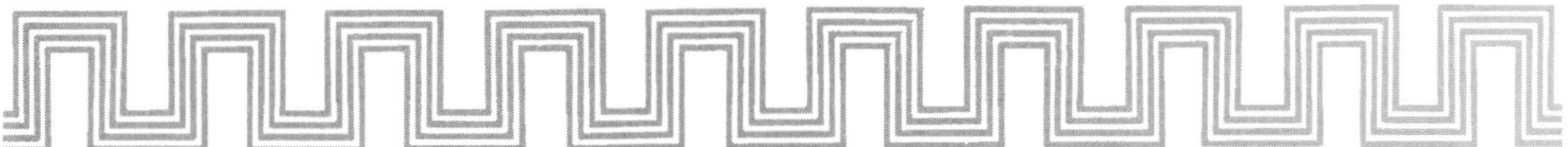

A Serial Story

Team up with a friend or two to write a story together.The two rules are:

1. Each person can write only one sentence at a time, and then he or she has to give the paper to the next person.
2. No one can kill off anyone else's characters.

Here is an example of the beginning of a serial story written by two people:

First person: The radio said that there was a hurricane coming.

Second person: They were evacuating our town.

First person: It was a good thing that my family and I were already ten miles away, going to visit my grandmother.

Second person: But then I remembered that our sick dog was home alone.

You can either continue working on this story or start another one of your own.

____

____

____

____

____

____

____

Name ______________________________ **Date** ________________

A VERY LONG EXCUSE

You have probably never done anything wrong. But if you had, wouldn't you like to be able to think of a really good excuse? Pretend, for example, that you traded the healthy lunch your mother gave you for a candy bar and soda, and your mother found out. You might want to explain with a story like the following:

> Well, see Mom, it's like this. I was really looking forward to the tofu salad sandwich, I really was. But I have this friend at school who is living with her aunt now, and her aunt won't give her any tofu. And she loves tofu. She needs tofu, because when she was little . . .

Either continue with this story or start your own.

____

____

____

____

____

____

____

____

____

Name ______________________________ **Date** ________________

Once you have several topics, write each one of them on a separate index card. Tell your students that one person will select a topic, and then everyone in the writing group will write on that topic for ten minutes. Students can be very nervous about this, because they are comfortable writing about only a few carefully chosen topics. In fact, this is the very reason you are introducing essay writing in this way. Tell your students that, in the future, teachers will probably ask them to write on a wide variety of subjects. This work will help free them up to do so.

Ask them to suggest a topic that they think you know nothing about. Once they have done so, model how you would handle this challenge. For example, if the subject is basketball, and you truly are not knowledgeable about the sport, you could write:

> Basketball is a sport. Really tall people run back and forth up and down the court trying to get the ball in the hoop. But I don't understand why they don't stop and congratulate themselves once they've made a basket. They just keep running up and down the court again.

The lightness of your approach is very important. Keep taking turns choosing those topics, and eventually your students will believe that they can write about just about anything. Once they have been writing for ten minutes, ask people to share their work. Allow them not to do so if they are reluctant, but encourage sharing; it's a great modeling time.

When students are comfortable with essays, introduce them to the following essay structure:

- An introductory paragraph tells what the essay is about.
- Supporting paragraphs express the thoughts and ideas in more detail.
- An ending paragraph draws conclusions.

This follows the basic paragraph structure. It helps students feel comfortable with longer essays.

WHAT TO DO ABOUT GRAMMAR

It's commonly understood that students with dyslexia often have difficulty with the mechanics of language, or grammar. Sometimes because of this, teachers focus on the weakness and have students complete page after page of exercise sheets. This is not an effective way to help students with dyslexia. They can complete numerous pages and still exhibit a lack of understanding about the grammar they have been "studying."

Following are three basic principles for effective grammar instruction:

1. **Keep it simple.** Limit the amount of information presented so that it can be easily incorporated into a student's work.

2. **Use multimodality and interactive games to teach grammar**. Students will be much more engaged and attentive.

3. **Practice a lot.**

CONCEPTS TO PRESENT

You want to give your students the sense that there is a logical order to the English language: Different types of words have certain purposes, there are rules for when to capitalize words, and there are other rules for adding punctuation marks to sentences.

The following is the suggested sequence for presenting grammar concepts:

1. A noun is a person, place, or thing.
2. A verb is an action word.
3. A sentence consists of a subject (who or what the sentence is about) and a predicate (tells what is happening or gives information about the subject).
4. Every sentence begins with a capital letter.
5. Every sentence ends with a punctuation mark.
6. An adjective is a word that describes a noun.
7. An adverb is a word that describes a verb.
8. There are words called pronouns, conjunctions, prepositions, and articles in the English language.
9. Quotation marks are used to separate spoken language from the rest of a sentence.
10. There are important places where you capitalize the first letter in a word, such as the first word of a sentence or a specific name of a person, place, or holiday.
11. Commas help represent a pause in spoken English.

The following examples of interactive activities help students with dyslexia really learn about grammar:

1. **Play the noun game.** Using index cards, students make a deck of at least 40 cards by writing one noun per card. Place the cards face down on the table. Depending on your students' level, ask them to select one to three cards and to orally make up a sentence using the nouns they have chosen. If they are able to do so, they keep the cards for the nouns they have been able to use. For advanced students, have them roll a die, so that they may be asked to make up a sentence using six different nouns. Students really enjoy this game and like to play it over and over.

2. **Play the Let's Talk game.** This activity helps students learn about quotation marks. Begin by saying a simple sentence like "I woke up late this morning." Write what you have just said on the board or on a large piece of paper and draw a circle around what you have said. Then, erase the circle, add quotation marks, and add "I said."

Next, ask one of your students to tell the group something in a simple sentence, and repeat the same procedure. When your students have mastered the simple sentence quote, practice with interrupted quotations.

EDITING

Students with dyslexia often have two different types of experiences with editing. In the first, someone takes a student's written work and types it, correcting all spelling and grammar errors with no consultation with the student. This does allow the student to feel a sense of pride in his work, but it doesn't teach him grammar. It also reinforces the idea that someone else has to intervene in order for his work to be really acceptable.

In the second, someone makes corrections on his written work (often in red) and hands it back to the student to copy. The second type of experience only reinforces the student's perception that he's not very good at writing.

Learning to self-edit should be an empowering and pleasurable experience. Students should feel that they are learning things about the language, and that they are getting better at finding and correcting their own mistakes. The two basic principles for teaching self-editing follow:

- Students should be held accountable only for the spelling and grammar issues that they are capable of recognizing and correcting.
- Editing should be learned in a sequential way.

This work can begin even at the word writing level. The following is a suggested sequence:

1. Begin by noticing individual words. Some are long, others are short. Some have endings, such as "ing."
2. Every sentence begins with a capital letter.
3. Every sentence ends with an ending punctuation mark.
4. There are conventional ways to spell words. Students should be held accountable only for spelling elements that they have completely mastered.
5. Most sentences, other than one word sentences like "Hi" need a subject and a predicate.

6. Quotation marks are used to separate spoken language from the rest of a sentence.
7. There are important places where you capitalize the first letter in a word, such as all the important words in book titles.
8. Commas help represent a pause in spoken English.
9. Written work of more than a few sentences should be divided into paragraphs.
10. Writing should be clear and not confusing.
11. Good transitions and organization are important for good writing.
12. One point of view is usually maintained consistently throughout a piece of writing.

With your student, select a short piece of his writing that you both will focus on. Ask him to read his work and to look for one very specific type of error. For example, ask him to check and see if all of his sentences begin with a capital letter. If your student finds any such errors, wait while he corrects them. Then ask, "Are you ready for me to be your editor?" If he is, read through the same selection and look for the same type of error. If you find some, put a light pencil checkmark in the left margin of the line where each error is located. Ask your student to read his work over again and to be especially aware of the lines that have checkmarks in the margin, because each checkmark indicates that one thing needs to be changed. Once your student has discovered his errors, wait while he corrects them. Then, ask him to erase the checkmarks.

Keep editing sessions short, not more than ten or fifteen minutes, and never point out more than a few errors for correction. Your goal is not a perfect product; it is much more process oriented. Your goal is to help your student begin to feel comfortable correcting his own work. You want him to feel that he *can* find his own mistakes and that, he *does* have the skills to correct them. At that point, he will begin to notice his own work much more and will take more care and pride in his writing.

OTHER WRITING OPPORTUNITIES

There is a wealth of enjoyable and exciting stimuli for creating good writing activities for the student with dyslexia. These provide excellent practice. Always remember the four basic principles:

- Ask students to write at or below their comfort level (word, sentence, paragraph, or multiparagraph).
- Structure the activity so that students know how to begin writing and how to continue on with the project.
- Make the activity relevant to their experiences.

- Make it fun.

Five types of stimuli, along with one specific activity for each one, are listed here to give a flavor of the types of things that can be done. All the different writing levels are represented.

Poetry

Write a first letter game poem. In this type of poem, a word or phrase is written vertically, one letter to a line. The poet then starts each line of his poem with the letter that is thus provided. Usually, the subject matter of the poem is determined by the stimulus word or phrase. For example, if a person named Samuel is writing such a poem based on his name, he could write:

Says what he thinks
Acts like a movie star, sometimes
Makes great pizza on Saturday nights for his friends
Understands a lot about life
Expects people to be honest
Likes most people he meets

Some good stimulus words and phrases are:

- A season of the year, like "Winter"
- A natural phenomenon, such as "A Tornado"
- The phrase "I wish"
- The phrase "In a Forest"

An independent activity sheet, "If I Were A Cat," which illustrates a first-letter game poem is provided on page 170.

Literature Connection

Write a "What Happens Next?" essay or story. Read a short story such as "Thank You, M'am" by Langston Hughes, which can be found in *Something in Common, and Other Stories* by Langston Hughes (American Century Series, Hill and Wang, 1963). This story tells of a boy who tries to steal a woman's purse. He doesn't succeed and, instead, gets caught by his intended victim, Mrs. Luella Bates Washington Jones. The reader knows that Mrs. Jones's kindness and common sense will have a great impact on the boy, but perhaps your students would like to think about that more deeply. Maybe they'd like to write a short essay about what they think will happen to the boy, or they can write an ending to the continuing story.

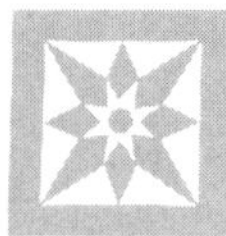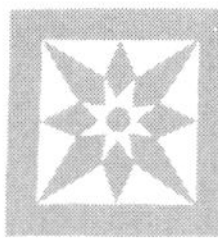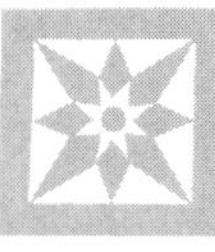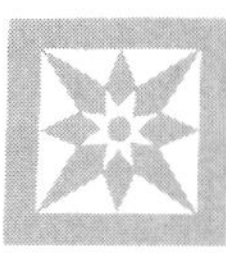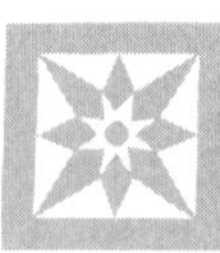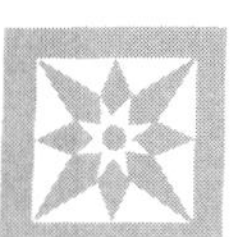

If I Were A Cat

Write an "If I Were a Cat" poem. Begin each line with the letter that is placed at the beginning. Try to think of things that you would really like to do if you could become a feline for a day. For example:

> If I were a cat,
> Fabulous tuna would fill my food bowl.
> I would pretend to take several naps
> While watching closely for any invading armies of mice.

I f I were a cat, ______________________

F ______________________

I ______________________

W ______________________

E ______________________

R ______________________

E ______________________

A ______________________

C ______________________

A ______________________

T ______________________

Name ______________________ **Date** ______________

HOLIDAYS

Create a special holiday. Some holidays have recently been created. For example, Kwanzaa was created in 1966 to call attention to the attributes of unity, sharing, responsibility, faith, talents, determination, and generosity in the African-American community.

If they wish, students can create a holiday of their own. This holiday can honor, for example, a special person, an animal or flower, or an event that is meaningful to them. As they create their holidays, they can consider questions like the following:

- What is the date or season of the holiday?
- Are there special rituals, such as the reading of poems?
- Do people gather together, or is the holiday celebrated privately?
- Are there special meals and foods?

WRITING LETTERS

Make and write a picture postcard. The U.S. Postal Service requires that a postcard be no smaller than $3^1/_2$ by 5 inches, and no larger than $4^1/_4$ by 6 inches. Four inch by six inch index cards, therefore, make excellent post cards. Students enjoy decorating the blank side with their own art work or with cut-out art from old magazines.

On the lined side, students can either write to their friends about their artistic creations or just send friendly greetings.

USING THE NEWSPAPER

Write descriptive words, sentences, or paragraphs about pictures from the newspaper. To present this activity, you need a collection of interesting newspaper photographs. For example, students love writing about the picture that shows a young man with a Mohawk haircut carrying a pet rat on his head. It helps some students to get started if you first brainstorm together for some good key words that come to mind as you look at the photograph. Record these key words on the chalkboard or on a piece of paper and let your students start writing.

A TYPICAL LESSON PLAN

A lesson is based on an hour and consists of four activities. The lesson is constructed in this way for the following reasons:

- Students with relatively short attention spans can be actively engaged throughout the entire lesson. There is less off-task behavior, because by the time they are thinking of focusing on something else, you are presenting another interesting activity.

- It is hard work for a student with dyslexia to work on writing. Varying types of activities, therefore, enables him to avoid developing too much fatigue.
- Several modalities can be utilized within one lesson.

If you do not have an hour for a lesson, still create your lesson plan based on that time. You can present sections of it in a sequential way, in other words, in either two half-hour sessions or even four fifteen minute sessions.

These are the four sections of the lesson:

1. **Writing lists**. Students begin by writing a list of something. Examples are
   - sports
   - toppings for pizza
   - clothing
   - forms of transportation
   - things that you can put on your feet
   - things you would take on a three-day camping trip
   - things that will make you happy

The variety of list topics is endless and should be chosen with your students' interests and writing levels in mind. List writing is a great way to begin a lesson, because it is nonthreatening and fun. Students enjoy this activity and it helps them to be immediately successful. It also provides essential practice in helping them to generate ideas and to put these ideas onto paper.

2. **The structured writing section.** This is where your students work directly on the basic forms of the written language. Choose among word writing, sentence writing, paragraph writing, or writing research reports, book reports, stories, or essays. All of these have been discussed previously.
3. **Learning some new skills and reinforcing others.** Two types of activities occur in this section of the lesson. In the first, grammar and editing concepts are introduced and worked with. In the second, the emphasis is on writing practice and motivation. Here, your students can write poetry or letters. They can use literature or the newspaper to help them generate writing ideas. Holidays can be a source of inspiration. All of these were discussed in the previous section.
4. **Listening to a teacher read a book.** At the end of each lesson, read from a favorite book for approximately ten minutes. To produce written language, you need a sense of it, so encourage your students to listen carefully by introducing conversation about the work being read.

   A major benefit of ending each lesson in this way is that it helps everyone relax. Students and teacher can enjoy a good book together. This not only helps to develop good relationships but it also helps students perceive writing instruction as something they can manage. It ends each writing session on a happy, positive note.

IMPORTANT CONSIDERATIONS

Writing Notebooks

Supply each student with a loose leaf three ring binder for writing instruction. The notebooks should be organized into sections, using tabs. For example, sections can include lists, sentences, paragraphs, writing poetry, and writing letters. In effect, a student's notebook will include whatever he is working on.

These notebooks are helpful because they provide one place where all writing work can be stored. After a student has worked on a paper, he can immediately file it in the appropriate section. This helps him learn how to organize his work. Because students with dyslexia also often have a tendency to lose things, it helps to avoid that whole issue. Your student can always feel proud that all his work is stored safely and neatly.

The second benefit of the writing notebook is that it serves as a record of your student's progress. Ask him to put a date on every page, and in a few weeks, he will be looking back and noticing how well he is progressing.

Writing with Your Students

It is very important to write on the same type of task while your students are working. In this way, you can model an effective way to approach the task. When sharing time comes, you can also model effective writing. Students with dyslexia need quiet, safe time to compose their thoughts and to risk putting them on paper. When you sit and write with them, you provide silent support for this process.

Sharing

It is best if all students share their work at every lesson. If a student is reluctant to share, you need to treat this with great care. You can ask your student if he would like you to read his work for him. If he remains hesitant, respect his wishes. Usually, once students realize that sharing is a safe time, in which writing efforts will always be treated respectfully, they are happy to share.

How to Praise

Unfortunately, many students with dyslexia have received what they consider false praise. They may have been told that they were doing a good job, when it was very clear that their work was not measuring up to the work of their peers.

Therefore, it can be most effective to respond to content, as opposed to just saying, "Fine job." For example, if a student has written a paragraph about border collies, you can say, "It's really interesting to me that you said that even border collie puppies will try to herd little animals, like kittens. That's amazing." When you respond in this way, you tell your student that you have really been listening to his writing. He has expressed very interesting information in an effective way. This response helps him feel more enthusiastic about picking up his pencil for the next written task.

PRIVACY ISSUES

Sometimes, a topic can be suggested that is not safe for your student to write about. For example, the topic might be to describe a meal students have shared with their families. Unfortunately, some students may have unhappy memories or other issues associated with eating with their families. Or they may not have a conventional family and may not want to disclose this information. Watch your students carefully. If they exhibit discomfort with a potentially troubling topic, simply say to them, "If you would like to write about something else, let's brainstorm for a minute about what that might be. Writing about a meal is only one idea. We can probably come up with a much better one."

SPELLING

Often, new writers are very concerned about their spelling and will stop themselves in the middle of the writing process to ask how to spell a word. Encourage your students to make good guesses and to write on. If a student is insistent, give him a written model of the requested word, but assure him that he will not be judged on his spelling. Tell him that, if he wishes, you will tell him how to spell any word he wants, once he finishes his writing, and he can correct any spelling errors at that point.

This approach helps students relax around the spelling issue when they write; thus, their writing fluency improves. They don't sit there thinking about how they can avoid writing words they don't know how to spell. Rather, they can focus on writing more freely because they know that they can deal with spelling issues later.

INTERVIEW WITH MIKE

Mike spoke in Chapter 6 about reading. Here, he talks about what writing was like for him before he received proper instruction as an adult.

What was it like for you when you were a kid, when you were asked to write something?

Well, I kept on writing about the same thing, over and over again.

What did you keep writing about?

I don't remember stories I wrote about, but I remember I used to write about the same thing.

Why did you do that?

Because it was easier.

Were you comfortable with the writing process?

No. It was drudgery. I knew what I wanted to say, but I couldn't get it down. I couldn't spell. I knew what I wrote, but other people couldn't understand what I wrote.

How old were you at that point?

Third or fourth grade.

What would they say to you, when they couldn't understand?

That's why I used to do the same thing over and over again.

You said that spelling was one of the problems. Was there another?

Speech. Pronouncing the words. Sometimes we had to take what we wrote down and say it in front of the class. Everybody knew I had a problem, pronouncing some words. But once I got going, I kind of made up the story. The teacher knew I was making it up.

The teacher was okay with that?

Sometimes she would stop me. Sometimes, she would let me keep going. It depended on how far off track I got. But the trouble is, I always had to pass it in. The story that I'd told and the one that I'd written down weren't the same thing.

What grade was that?

Fifth grade, something like that.

So the main impediments were the spelling, getting it down. How about forming the letters? Were you able to do that okay?

Well, I never seemed . . . I never thought I had a hard time writing, but as I got older, I recognized that I wasn't writing as clear. But I used to write sloppy, just to cover up what I was writing.

Oh, you'd cover up words that you didn't know how to spell?

Yes. I always thought that my handwriting was good.

In high school, what would you do if you had to write a report?

It would take me hours to write a report.

How many hours would it take you to do a one- or two-page report?

Probably eight hours. That's why I couldn't see how people could go to college, with all that writing. It would take me days to do all that stuff.

But you've gone to college.

But that was years after. See, when I was in high school, I took all lower level classes, so there weren't a lot of writing requirements. There are college prep classes and then there are general classes, and then there are classes under that. That's basically where I was.

When you got to college, you were able to cope with writing demands.

Yeah, but it took—it just took me such a long time. First, I had to read it, which took a long time, and then write about it, which took longer. It took me two or three drafts. By that time, the computer came along.

So that made it easier.

Yes, it made it a lot easier.

You're a good writer now. What are some of the things that have helped you?

Just learning how to spell some of the words. Instead of skipping over words, I write the words I really want to say. Before, if I didn't know how to spell something, I'd sidetrack it somehow. I'd just try to use another word that I knew how to spell, which ended up being a simpler word. Or I'd lengthen out the sentence, which actually was a good thing, because it stretched it out. That's what I always used to get inked for, the shortness of sentences.

So you used to skip over a word that you couldn't spell. But that broke your train of thought.

Yes. That's exactly what happened. You try to take and skip around, and you lose the whole theme of what you're trying to say. And before, I didn't know how to form papers. I didn't know about the introduction and the main body and the conclusion. I didn't know how to do all that.

How do you feel about your capabilities now, as a writer?

I'm okay. I don't think I'm the greatest. I've been noticing more, I've been catching that I don't write what I want to say. I know what I want to say, but my mind's having me write down something else, different words. Or I'll leave out words. I'll be going along, and I'll just skip over a word. My mind thinks it's there, but it's not on the paper. That happens a lot.

Is there anything else that you want to say about your experiences with writing?

I had this writing class in college; you had to describe stuff. Once, we had to describe how we drove to the college. That was pretty easy. I had something that I could just tell about. That was easy. But if I had to take and make up a route, that would have taken me hours to do. And then, if I had to do research, it was hard to take that and put it all together.

Chapter 10

TEACHING MATH

Some students with dyslexia easily learn mathematics with traditional curriculum, but many do not. These students do not necessarily have dyscalculia, the neurologically based difficulty with calculation; very few people have this particular neurological issue. Many students with dyslexia, however, have difficulty with math. The learning style issues that affect their acquisition of language and concepts in other academic areas can also affect their learning in math. They can have difficulty with:

- the language of mathematics
- the written output required, such as with writing numbers
- the visual-motor skill required to copy arithmetic problems from the board and other places
- the spatial abilities required to complete complex calculation problems
- the short-term and long-term memories required to remember arithmetic facts
- visualizing mathematical concepts that are presented only in two-dimensional (paper and pencil) form

It is also true that students with dyslexia often have the cognitive capacity and insight to become gifted mathematicians if they are not stopped in their tracks by early difficulty with inappropriate instruction. Think for a moment about Albert Einstein, who frequently got into trouble for making errors with arithmetic calculations during his early school days. At that time, his special abilities in math were not noticed, because he was unable to give the quick, rote, accurate answers that his teachers desired. Fortunately, he did not let this early "failure" stop his intellectual interest in the field.

WHAT IS APPROPRIATE INSTRUCTION?

Given the difficulties that students with dyslexia often experience with math, what, then, is appropriate instruction? How can we help our students to become competent, and even gifted, mathematicians? Basic principles still apply:

- ***Use Multimodality Instruction.*** Introduce concepts with concrete objects and spend a great deal of the learning time with them. Move to a two-dimensional presentation only when students are very firm in their knowledge of the concept being studied. The two-dimensional presentation should be in the following order:
    1. Pictorial, in which students use pictures without concrete objects
    2. Abstract symbols such as numerals, signs, and equations
- ***Use the Experiential, Interactive Approach.*** Students are active learners who experiment with concrete objects to discover concepts and math facts.
- ***Ask Students to Verbalize what They Are Discovering in Their Own Words.*** This provides important feedback, especially with developing memory for math facts.
- ***Be a Team.*** Students and you, as members of this learning team, will look for solutions to problems.
- ***Present Material in Small Steps.***
- ***Present Material Sequentially.***
- ***Review and Practice in Every Lesson.***

The subject of math covers a sizable amount of content. For the purposes of this text, we will focus primarily on arithmetic, that problematic area with which students with dyslexia so frequently have difficulty. Arithmetic involves knowing number concepts, or what abstract numbers represent. It also involves being able to manipulate those numbers: adding, subtracting, multiplying, and dividing. A solid foundation in arithmetic is essential for successful learning in mathematics.

Later in this chapter, recommended resources are offered for further study of some different and other more advanced areas of math. The math issues involved in using money and telling time will be discussed in Chapter 12, "Teaching Everyday Skills."

BEFORE NUMBERS: BEGINNING THE WORK

The most basic thing that students need is the understanding that each written number represents a quantity, and each number is unique. Furthermore, these numbers relate to one another.

Some students need preliminary work before they begin the process of acquiring these understandings, however. For example, they need to become adept at observing their environment and at noticing the dimensions of things, like size and quantity. Do things match? Are they the same or different? Are there recurring patterns of color or shape that can be observed? Dr. Maria Montessori suggests interesting activities that help develop awareness and good observation skills. In one of her activities, for example, children are given ten rods, all of a different length. The first one is a "one" size, and the others each lengthen by a "one" rod. The longest is therefore a "ten." No number language is used, but children are encouraged to arrange these rods in a row from shorter to taller, thus creating a stair. Public libraries usually have books by Dr. Montessori and, also, books about the method. Two such resources are *A Montessori Handbook, "Dr. Montessori's Own Handbook" with Additional New Material on Current Montessori Theory and Practice*, edited by R. C. Orem (G.P. Putnam's Sons, 1965) and *Basic Montessori: Learning Activities for Under-Fives* by David Gettman (St. Martin's Press, 1987).

TEACHING ARITHMETIC

The *Structural Arithmetic*[1] program by Catherine Stern, Margaret B. Stern, and Toni S. Gould (Educators Publishing Service, 1992) offers an interesting and effective approach for students with dyslexia. It provides instruction for the four computation procedures of addition, subtraction, multiplication, and division. Even though it is primarily designed for preschool through grade 4, it can, with appropriate modifications, be used for older students. In fact, it's recommended that you carefully assess your older student's knowledge of these basic skills. Many older students with dyslexia have been "getting by" with great effort and scattered rote learning. When you really check, you may discover that they are, in fact, missing some critical understandings.

The basic tenets of *Structural Arithmetic* are:

- The goal of the program is to help students learn to reason by themselves. This emphasis on the development of cognitive ability utilizes experiments, rather than rote learning.
- Students learn facts in groups rather than in isolation. In the latter, for example, students are often given two sets of tangible objects, such as beads, and told to count all of them, as with 6 + 3 = 9. This does introduce them to that particular fact, but it does not help them discover its relationship to other facts.
- Math facts are presented visually, as opposed to by counting. For example, when a student is asked to add 3 + 2, she is given materials that she can manipulate and measure in a number track, rather than just saying "3, 4, 5." The latter can make little sense to the student, because counting really is rote repeating of words. She can also make many errors with the counting system, especially if the sum is a number in the teens.

[1] Catherine Stern, Margaret B. Stern, and Toni S. Gould (Educators Publishing Service, © 1992). Used by permission.

- Students are encouraged to experiment with materials in ways that help develop their logical, spatial reasoning skills.
- Students are encouraged to verbally express the math concepts and facts that they have been discovering. This verbalization provides important feedback and helps them retain information.
- Emphasis is placed on developing relationships among facts, so that students don't have to memorize so many of them.
- Most instructional work is interactive. Workbooks are presented only after concepts and facts are very familiar, and they are used only in a role that is supportive to the main work with the teacher.
- Teachers are careful to notice if students are understanding directions and other verbal interactions.

To gain a sense of this program's approach, the following games and activities from it are briefly described below.

LEARNING NUMBER NAMES

Play a game *Structural Arithmetic* calls *The Snake Game.*[2] Number markers from one to ten are provided, as well as ten groups of blocks, representing the numbers from one to ten. The "one" block has one block, the "two" block has two, which are joined together, and so on. The multiples are all joined. In this program, the blocks are referred to as number blocks.

Form two teams and have the first player select a number marker out of the several that have been placed face down on a tray. The student then finds the one block or connected blocks that represent that number and starts a "snake." Players take turns selecting cards and adding to their team's "snake."

ADDITION

For this activity, the 10-box is used.[3] It is a square box with room for ten rectangles of ten blocks each. Select two number blocks that, together, make a ten; for example, 2 + 8. As you place these in the number box, say, "The 2 needs the 8 in order to be a 10." Next, ask the students to make some other combinations that together make 10. Ask them to say what they are doing in their own words.

Show models of the "plus" and "equal" signs. Then, show the students how to record a number fact with paper and pencil. They write the fact they have just represented with number blocks, and then they say it.

---

[2] *The Snake Game* is from *Structural Arithmetic II* by Margaret Stern and Toni S. Gould (Educators Publishing Service, © 1990). Used by permission.

[3] This activity is from *Structural Arithmetic I* by Margaret Stern, and Toni S. Gould (Educators Publishing Service, © 1988). Used by permission.

SUBTRACTION

Play a game *Structural Arithmetic* calls *The Scarf Game.*[4] For this activity, you need the 10-box, number blocks from 1 to 10, and a scarf. Place the number blocks on the table in front of your students. Ask your students to close their eyes, and then hide two blocks that make 10 under the scarf. When they open their eyes, show them one of the blocks, for example, a 6. Ask them to tell you how many blocks will be left if you take away this 6. Once they have stated "4," remove the scarf to check. Ask students to verbalize the fact 10 - 6 = 4.

MULTIPLICATION

In the *Structural Arithmetic III*,[5] multiplication is presented as a unique way of dealing with numbers, as opposed to presenting it as relating to addition, as in $3 \times 2 = 2 + 2 + 2$. Rather, multiplication involves taking a named amount more than once. Thus, in the above-named equation, the student would select a 2 number block three times and then measure these in a number track, a long rectangle with an indented track into which the number blocks fit. This program is also unique in that it doesn't present the multiplication tables in order but starts with 10, then 1, 2, 5, and 9 (because it is so close in quantity to 10).

To introduce the 10 table in *Structural Arithmetic III*,[6] a material called the dual board is used. It is a square block that has parallel rectangles into which number blocks of 10 each can be placed. On the bottom of the board, the single digits of 1 to 10 are recorded, thus recording the number of tens. On the top, the numbers 10, 20, 30, and so forth, are placed. Students are asked to place one number block of ten in the board and are shown how to record $1 \times 10 = 10$. They are then asked to place more groups of tens in the board, such as 4 groups, and then record the fact, $4 \times 10 = 40$. Students discover and record all of the other facts in the ten table in that manner.

DIVISION

All of the multiplication tables are learned thoroughly before division is introduced. This helps avoid confusion between the two. Also, students with dyscalculia can have unique problems with division. A major one is the confusion with the physical structure of the written division problem. For example, the written problems they have worked on for addition, subtraction, and multiplication all have the numbers to be dealt with above the line, and the answer is below, as in

$$\begin{array}{r} 3 \\ \underline{+\,2} \end{array} \qquad \begin{array}{r} 8 \\ \underline{-\,4} \end{array} \qquad \begin{array}{r} 6 \\ \underline{\times 7} \end{array}$$

---

[4] This game is from *Structural Arithmetic II* by Margaret Stern and Toni S. Gould (Educators Publishing Service, © 1990). Used by permission.

[5] Margaret Stern and Toni S. Gould (Educators Publishing Service, © 1992). Used by permission.

[6] Margaret Stern and Toni S. Gould (Educators Publishing Service, © 1992). Used by permission.

The very shape of the division problem, with its long line and curve can make them unable to understand what they should do. The following activity can help with this.

Play a game that *Structural Arithmetic* calls *Under the Box.*[7] It utilizes a number track. The game also uses some number blocks and a small box.

If, for example, you are working on the problem 35 divided by 5, show your students ten 5 blocks, the number track, and the box. Ask your students to close their eyes, and then cover up seven of the 5 blocks. Tell your students to open their eyes, and then tell them that the blocks under the box measure up to 35 in the number track. Ask them how many number blocks of 5 will be under the box. When they are able to say the correct answer, ask them to record the fact in a division formula. This activity helps students to visualize that the number of blocks under the box corresponds to the number "under the line" of a division problem.

The *Structural Arithmetic* program covers all the major aspects of computational work, including writing the numerals; regrouping with addition, subtraction, and multiplication; division with remainders; and adding with fractions. In addition, it deals with important everyday mathematical challenges such as volume measures, telling time, and money. There are also suggestions for word problem work.

BEYOND COMPUTATION

Once students have mastered the basic concepts involved with the four processes of number calculation and have developed enough memory of rote facts to help them use these concepts with facility, it's time to move on to other work. There are so many things to be learned: patterns, graphing, determining averages, working with decimals, working with fractions and percent, and so on. To avoid confusion in the great mass of data and concepts that are important in the mathematical world, it is helpful to have a published program that defines a sequence of how concepts will be presented. The following programs all offer interesting learning opportunities for the student with dyslexia.

On Cloud Nine: Visualizing and Verbalizing for Math by Kimberly Tuley and Nanci Bell (Gander Publishing, 1997) is based on the same concepts that the *Structural Arithmetic* program advocates; however, it adds another step. The authors believe that it is critical for students to be able to form mental images of math concepts. They therefore introduce concepts with manipulatives, as does *Structural Arithmetic*, but they then make sure that the students are able to visualize and verbalize these ideas. Then, computation is introduced. An important factor when you consider this program is to be aware of the authors' recommendation that students begin instruction with *Visualizing and Verbalizing for*

[7] This game is from *Structured Arithmetic III* by Margaret Stern and Toni S. Gould (Educators Publishing Service, © 1992). Used by permission.

Language Comprehension and Thinking by Nanci Bell (Academy of Reading Publications, 1986, 1991). This program purports that people need to create mental pictures in their minds to be able to understand language. In a careful sequence of instruction, students are taught how to create these pictures. *On Cloud Nine*, therefore, requires a significant commitment. It can, however, be an important resource for the student who is experiencing serious difficulty with math concepts.

Attack Math: Arithmetic Tasks to Advance Computational Knowledge by Carole Greenes, George Immerzeel, Linda Schulman, and Rika Spungin (Educators Publishing Service, 1985) offers three workbooks in each computational area. It covers grades 1–6. Even though workbooks are not used as the primary program for the student with dyslexia, these books offer good supplementary materials with which students can practice. The number of computation problems or word problems is limited on each page. This makes the books manageable for the student with dyslexia.

Mathematics Their Way by Mary Baretta-Lorton (Addison-Wesley, 1976) is a wonderful program that is a lot of fun for students. A real advantage of this program is that readily available materials are used in the activities. This program is intended for grades K–2 and covers areas such as logical thinking, graphing, and sorting and classifying. Because the program does not obviously "look" like a primary level resource, it can be used for older students with dyslexia, if they need this level of work.

Mathematics: A Way of Thinking by Robert Baretta-Lorton (Addison-Wesley, 1977) also offers hands-on discovery opportunities. This program has a similar philosophy to *Mathematics Their Way* and is intended for grades 3–6. As with the former program, it can easily be used for older students with dyslexia.

The Kim Marshall Series: Math, Parts A and B by Kim Marshall (Educators Publishing Service, *Part A*: 1982, 1984, 1997; *Part B*: 1983) is a program of two books that offer 35 cumulative units. These books are good for the more advanced student who can work somewhat independently. It covers concepts such as prime factors, rounding off numbers, metric measurement, and working with fractions.

OTHER SUPPLEMENTARY RESOURCES

A wealth of good books offer interesting interactive ideas for supporting work in math. Other books share historical information about the subject. Public libraries often have a selection of these books. Look up mathematics in the subject file, either in the card file or on computer, and see what your library has purchased. Some good resources are listed on the following page.

- *Family Math* by Jean Kerr Stenmark, Virginia Thompson and Ruth Cossey, illustrated by Marilyn Hill (The Lawrence Hall of Science, 1986 by the Regents, University of California).
- *The I Hate Mathematics Book* by Marilyn Burns (Little, Brown and Company, 1975).
- *Math for Every Kid: Easy Activities That Make Learning Math Fun* by Janice Van Cleaver (John Wiley and Sons, Inc., 1991).
- *Games for Math: Playful Ways to Help Your Child Learn Math, from Kindergarten to Third Grade*, written by Peggy Kaye with illustrations by the author (Pantheon Books, 1987).
- *Math Fun with Money Puzzlers* by Rose Wyler and Mary Elting, illustrated by Patrick Girouard (Julian Messner, 1992).
- *How to Count Like a Martian* by Glory St. John, (Henry Z. Walck, 1975).

A WORD ON USING MANIPULATIVES

Some teachers choose to make their own manipulatives rather than to purchase them. You can also use common, everyday objects like paper clips, buttons, or beans. Another option is to buy Unifix® cubes (interlocking cubes), number tracks, and other materials from a variety of suppliers. There is no magic to the manipulatives you choose to utilize. Two factors are important:

1. The manipulatives should be age appropriate for students.
2. A student should be looking at only one variable at a time; for example, if the student is using blocks to study number concepts, all the blocks in a given number set should be the same color. Blocks in a different number set can be a different color. Therefore, the student will easily be able to select one number group of red blocks and add this to another number set of yellow blocks.

EVERYDAY MATH

Students with dyslexia are usually practical people, and they appreciate learning about what is happening in their lives. Therefore, keep on the lookout for math opportunities during the day

For example, at one school, a teacher lives on a farm, where she has a few chickens. She sells her extra eggs at a local food co-op. The students are interested in this business because every spring, they help hatch chicks as a school project. And look at the opportunities for learning:

- Making a list of the cost of chicken feed and other expenses, and adding them up
- Figuring out how much profit is gained for every dozen eggs sold

- Figuring out how much money the co-op owes the teacher (number of dozens of eggs times price per dozen)

Opportunities to connect real life and math can also be simple and quick, and can occur at the most basic levels. For example, right before lunch, ask how many people have cold sandwiches and how many people will eat something hot. Count and record each number. Then, ask your students which group is larger. This type of interaction, geared to the math levels and interests of your students can be an important and effective way to reinforce math learning.

LITERATURE AND MATH

Literature also offers many fun and interesting opportunities for learning math. While you are reading a picture book to your students, for example, you can initiate conversation using math vocabulary and concepts, such as:

- Counting (For example, "How many elephants are there on that page?")
- Weight (For example, "What do you think is heavier, the piano or the lamp?")
- Measurement (For example, "How long do you think that table is?")

This doesn't have to be difficult to do. Just keep in mind the concepts that your students are studying, and look for places where you can discuss these concepts using books. Do this lightly and with no pressure, and your students will enjoy the intellectual challenge of it.

There are also some books that focus more directly on math concepts. Some good ones are the following:

How Much Is a Million? by David M. Schwartz, pictures by Steven Kellogg (Lothrop, Lee and Shepard, (1985).

Counting on Frank, written and illustrated by Rod Clement (Gareth Stevens Children's Books, 1991).

Each Orange Had 8 Slices by Paul Giganti, Jr., pictures by Donald Crews (Greenwillow Books, 1992).

Counting on the Woods, a poem by George Ella Lyon, photographs by Ann W. Olson (A DK Ink Book, 1998).

Eating Fractions by Bruce McMillan (Scholastic, Inc., 1991).

The book *Math Through Children's Literature: Making the NCTM Standards Come Alive* by Kathryn L. Braddon, Nancy J. Hall, and Dale Taylor (Teacher Ideas Press, 1993) lists many other good books. This resource also offers specific activities for the classroom.

A WORD ABOUT CALCULATORS

Calculators are a great tool, but they are no substitute for real learning. Students with dyslexia *can* learn math concepts and math facts. It requires appropriate instruction and hard work, but they can be successful, and they then can feel the great satisfaction that comes with this accomplishment. They, also, do not need to be dependent upon a technical support. Thus, they don't have to be afraid of being embarrassed in social situations in which basic math skills are required.

Calculators can be very helpful to check answers or to perform calculations in cases in which speed is required. They are a tool, and as with all tools, they can be extremely helpful when used appropriately.

INDEPENDENT ACTIVITY SHEETS

Use work sheets only to reinforce concepts and facts that have already been learned. Use them as supplementary materials for review and practice. Four good basic principles follow:

1. **It's best to make them yourself.** If you do this, you know that your student can succeed with all the problems on the page. Making them yourself also allows you to take your student's visual motor abilities and spatial skills into account, as well as her level of mathematics knowledge. Some students, for example, profit from having their independent work written on half inch or three-quarter inch graph paper. Two independent activity sheets, both titled "My Work," provide these grids on pages 191 and 192. See the samples of completed work on these grids, which precede the blank grids. Also, concerning word problems, if you write them yourself, you can relate the problems directly to your student's life, using names of friends and real-life situations.

2. **Keep the calculation and word problems simple.** What needs to be done should be easy to discern. Also, there should be very little distracting visual stimuli on the page. Six independent activity sheets are offered on pages 193–198 to illustrate these points, and it's suggested that you model your own work sheets on them. As students gain proficiency and confidence, you can place more problems on each page. They are as follows:

   - "Addition": provides problems with two-digit addition with no regrouping
   - "Subtraction": provides problems with two-digit subtraction with no regrouping
   - "Multiplication": provides problems with two-digit multiplication with no regrouping
   - "Division": provides problems with simple division
   - "Figure It Out with Addition or Subtraction": provides word problems involving addition and subtraction
   - "Figure It Out with Multiplication or Division": provides word problems involving multiplication and division.

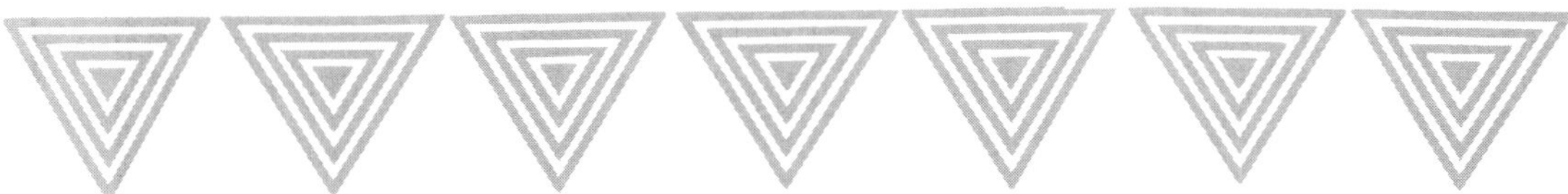

My Work

	4	2		6	5		
	+1	1		+2	4		
	5	3		8	9		
	3	7		1	6		
	+4	0		+2	3		
	7	7		3	9		

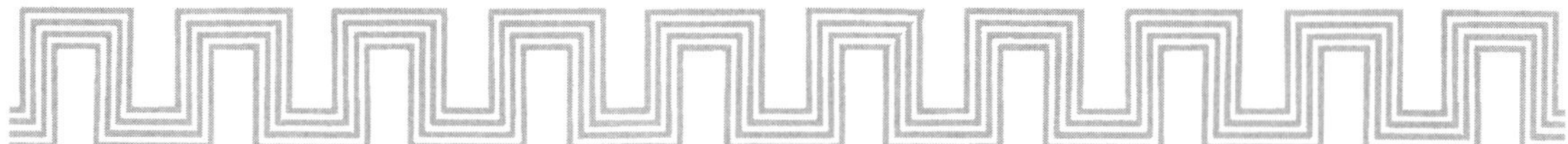

My Work

93	68	47
+12	–35	–23
81	33	24

58	35	28
+47	–14	–22
11	21	06

84	75	56
+53	–61	–43
31	14	13

My Work (I)

Name ______________________________ **Date** ________________

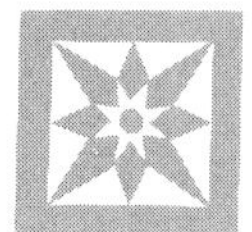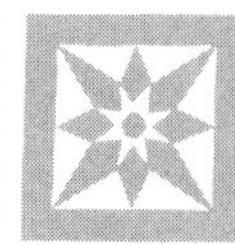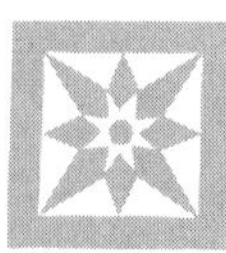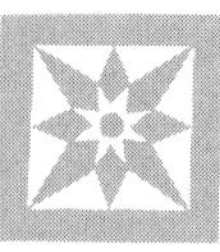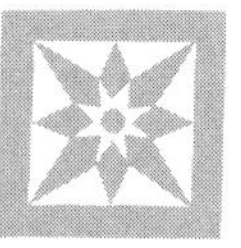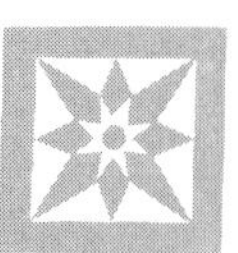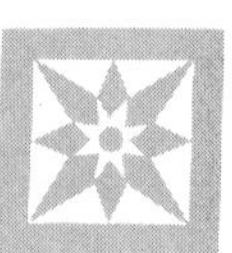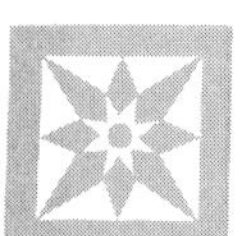

My Work (II)

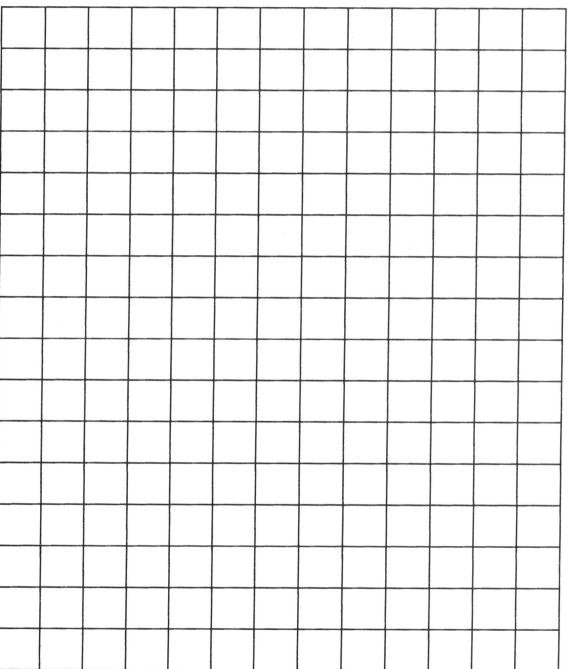

Name ______________________________ **Date** ________________

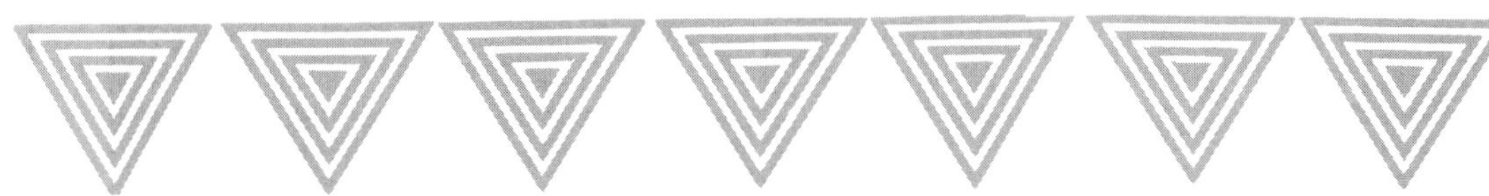

ADDITION

23 + 51	62 + 37	25 + 44
18 + 61	13 + 46	39 + 40
78 + 21	84 + 15	63 + 35

Name ______________________________ Date ________________

SUBTRACTION

57 − 11	63 − 32	78 − 45
31 − 10	49 − 27	86 − 53
99 − 65	26 − 14	38 − 24

Name ______________________ Date ______________

MULTIPLICATION

$$\begin{array}{r} 71 \\ \times\ 14 \\ \hline \end{array}$$

$$\begin{array}{r} 23 \\ \times\ 22 \\ \hline \end{array}$$

$$\begin{array}{r} 82 \\ \times\ 14 \\ \hline \end{array}$$

$$\begin{array}{r} 54 \\ \times\ 12 \\ \hline \end{array}$$

$$\begin{array}{r} 67 \\ \times\ 11 \\ \hline \end{array}$$

$$\begin{array}{r} 53 \\ \times\ 33 \\ \hline \end{array}$$

$$\begin{array}{r} 81 \\ \times\ 67 \\ \hline \end{array}$$

$$\begin{array}{r} 14 \\ \times\ 22 \\ \hline \end{array}$$

$$\begin{array}{r} 34 \\ \times\ 12 \\ \hline \end{array}$$

Name ______________________________ **Date** ________________

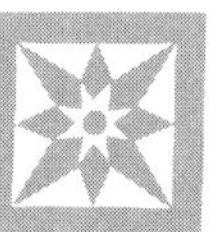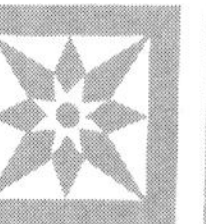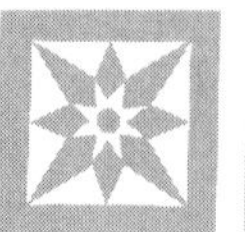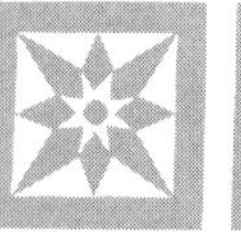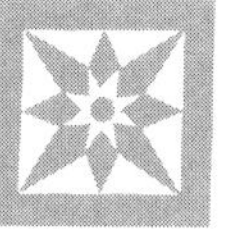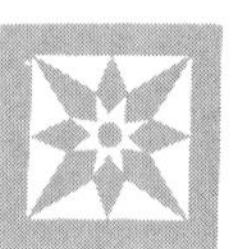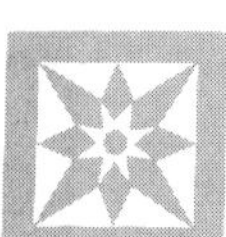

DIVISION

$5\overline{)45}$ $3\overline{)12}$ $6\overline{)30}$

$2\overline{)8}$ $7\overline{)42}$ $10\overline{)50}$

$8\overline{)48}$ $1\overline{)3}$ $9\overline{)18}$

Name ______________________ Date ______________

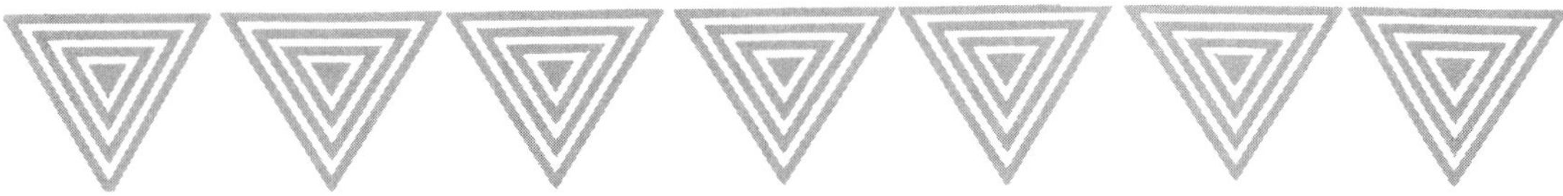

Figure It Out with Addition or Subtraction

First, make a drawing of the word problem. Then, use a number to answer the question.

Michael had 14 potato chips in a bag. He ate 6 of them. How many chips did he have left?

Answer: __________

Juanita found 2 pencils on Monday. On Tuesday, she found 3 more. How many pencils did Juanita find altogether?

Answer: __________

Name ________________________________ **Date** __________________

Figure It Out with Multiplication or Division

First, make a drawing to answer the word problem. Then, answer the question with a number.

Everyday, Kim rides 6 miles on a bus to get back and forth to school. How many miles does Kim ride the bus on 5 school days?

Answer: __________

Ebon made a pizza and cut it into 8 slices. He shared it equally with his sister. How many slices did Ebon and his sister each get?

Answer: __________

Name ________________________________ **Date** __________________

3. **Students should succeed with independent activity sheets.** If a student is not able to perform at least at 85 percent accuracy, the sheet is too hard and should simply be removed from her sight without comment. Or you can say,"Oh, I'm sorry that I made a mistake giving you that work. Here, try this one." Replace the sheet with a more appropriate one.

4. **Help students to discover any errors.** Say things like,"Why don't you check that one again?" That is much more empowering than an ugly correction mark. Students generally want to get their problems right, and they will develop careful habits from success and encouragement, not from pages and pages of corrected errors. The latter often make them give up, and they become unmotivated and sloppy.

If there is writing on the independent activity sheet for directions or for the word problems, make sure that students can read the text easily.

If, because of time issues, you decide to use published independent activity sheet programs, try to select work sheets that are simple and that have only a few visual elements on a page. As mentioned earlier in this chapter, *Attack Math* is a good supplementary workbook series. For some students who can be overwhelmed by a whole book, it is helpful to take individual sheets out of the workbooks and present them sequentially. *And this rule still applies:* Be careful that your student is highly successful on every page. If she is not, select other independent work for her.

Three independent activity sheets, described here, are fun for students to do; they are provided on pages 200–202.

- "Draw Me": This sheet requires students to represent numbers pictorially. This type of work sheet is simple and easy to prepare, and students who are working with number concepts enjoy the challenge.
- "Addition Bingo": This sheet offers a game in which students randomly write down numbers from 1 through 12 in the provided grid, and then play a game with a set of dice, in which they add the two numbers rolled. It gives them enjoyable practice with writing numbers and with addition.
- "Multiplication Bingo": This sheet offers a game in which students write multiples in boxes in the provided grid. They then roll two die and multiply the two numbers. It they have such a number on their grid, they color it in. The first player who has a completed row—vertical, horizontal, or diagonal—wins. And students always win, because they're practicing those multiplication facts.

DRAW ME

Draw six cats.

Draw five trees.

Draw three books.

Name ______________________ **Date** ______________

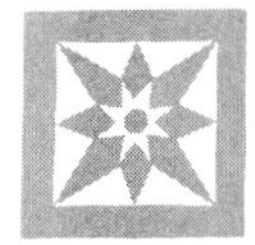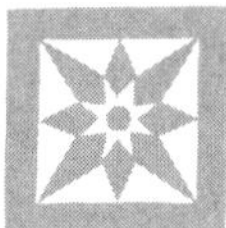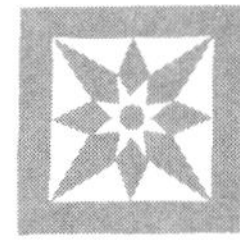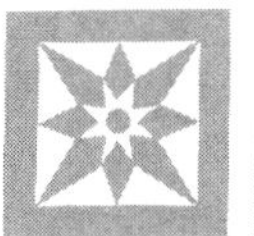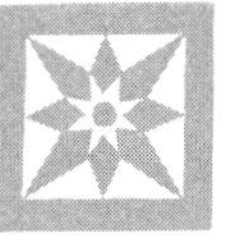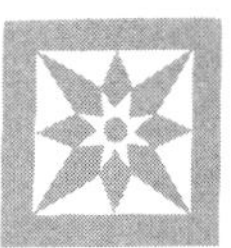

ADDITION BINGO

Find a friend or two and play Addition Bingo. First, write a number from 2 through 12 in each square, like the 3 that has been done for you. Then, roll two die and add up the number you get. If you have that number on your card, color one of those squares. The first person who colors a row wins the game.

3						

Name ______________________ **Date** ______________

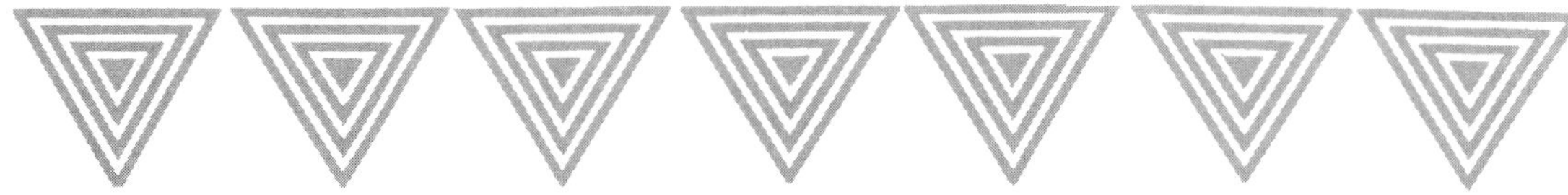

Multiplication Bingo

Find a friend or two and play Multiplication Bingo. First, fill each square below with one of the following numbers:

1, 2, 3, 4, 5, 6, 8, 9, 10, 12, 15, 16, 18, 20, 24, 25, 30, 36.

Then, roll two die and multiply the numbers. If you have that number on one of your grids, color it in. The first person to cover a row wins the game.

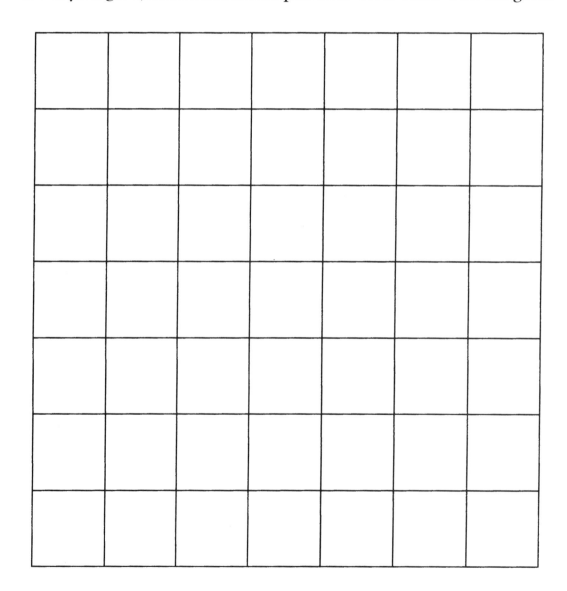

Name ______________________________ **Date** ________________

Interview with Sonia

Sonia is a gifted teacher who has taught students with dyslexia for over 30 years. Here, she speaks about effective methods for teaching math.

What are some of the basic principles for teaching math to students with dyslexia?

Use manipulatives. They have to touch, feel, and see in order to learn concepts. Start with three dimensional and then go to two dimensional, paper and pencil. Without that, don't bother to teach math.

Never, ever stop reviewing. Build a solid foundation and then build on top of it. Don't assume that they know anything, just because you've covered it. The biggest error that teachers make is assuming that the kids know it just because they know it today. Then they (teachers) hurry on and go to something else. It's a fine line between making sure they're being challenged and not overwhelming them by giving them something that's too difficult. It's better to err on the side of too easy. Kids get easily discouraged, and that's it, they're under the table.

You want hands-on, practical math. Many teachers make errors with manipulatives. They show the manipulatives to the kids, and then give them some problems to solve and tell them to go do the problems independently. Never give manipulatives for independent work unless they ask for them. Some kids, if they're older, can be embarrassed by them. Manipulatives are to be used <u>with</u> the teacher, and used properly. You'd better know how to use them and you'd better be excited about them.

What about multiplication tables? Have your students been successful learning those?

The myth is that students with dyslexia will never, ever learn their multiplication tables because they have short-term and long-term memory issues. It takes time and lots of review, but they get it. Practice every day.

It's a mistake to teach multiplication and division together. Multiplication should be taught to mastery, first. Otherwise, they get completely confused. They have to be solid with multiplication. Introduce it with manipulatives, and then go to two dimensional. Keep practicing every day.

How do you feel about students using calculators?

Don't use calculators, first of all because our kids punch in the wrong numbers. Calculators are okay for advanced students, only to check their work, but they don't teach basic concepts. You've got to know math so well, you can tell if an answer or calculation is plausible. You first have to know basic math well in order to use calculators.

CHAPTER 11

TEACHING RELATED SUBJECTS

Dyslexia can affect many areas of language, and thus it can have an impact on all subject areas. In addition, there are the other characteristics that can accompany dyslexia, like ADHD and difficulty with organizational skills. To make things more complicated, most students with dyslexia receive their instruction in the areas of social studies, science, physical education, music, and art in large classroom situations where the majority of learners have a traditional learning style. It is therefore very important to keep in mind the special needs and the special gifts of the student with dyslexia. If the learning style of these students is taken into consideration, they can flourish in these subject areas. They can think creatively, analyze patterns, and contribute a lot to the total classroom experience.

When teaching any subject, teachers must be aware of the following:

- how to present information
- how to help students interact with information
- how to evaluate acquisition of information

In all these areas, think back to the ten general principles of instruction discussed in detail in Chapter 5:

1. Involve the student.
2. Use multisensory teaching methods.
3. Teach students to use logic rather than rote memory.
4. Present material sequentially.
5. Present material in small units.
6. Practice, practice, practice, and review.
7. Help students organize time and space.
8. Individualize instruction.
9. Always be aware of the emotional climate.
10. Laugh a lot.

At first glance, this list may seem overwhelming, especially in a busy classroom where many students need attention and care. A teacher might ask, for example, "How can I individualize instruction when I have 25 students in my class?" In the following, we will first revisit all of the general principles, looking at how they can be applied to large class situations. Then, we will briefly discuss each subject area and give some suggestions for effective teaching. At the end of the chapter, the topics of homework and assessment will be addressed.

THE TEN GENERAL PRINCIPLES

INVOLVE THE STUDENT

Students with dyslexia tend to do better when they feel a sense of caring from their teachers. This is probably true of all students, but it is particularly so for people who have experienced failure in academic settings. Often, the student with dyslexia approaches a classroom setting the way a soldier approaches a field of land mines. There could be places for embarrassment everywhere. What if the teacher asks him to read some text aloud? In music, will he have to read the words of songs? What if he will be expected to memorize large quantities of data? Will spelling be counted on written work? What about tests? Will he have to write long essays with perfect spelling and grammar? In physical education, will he be put on teams where he has to perform well individually to help his team succeed?

It is recommended that these issues be addressed early, so that the student can relax. If expectations are higher than a student can meet (excellent spelling, for example), modifications of expectations or strategies for appropriate support must be planned.

Create a private conference time and talk about concerns. Also discuss goals, both yours and the student's, so that both of you can feel that you are forming a learning team. Three reproducibles are provided on pages 207–210: "Finding Out About Learning Style," "My Learning Style" (for the student) and "A Learning Contract." These pages will help you establish your "learning team" with your student. They can begin and focus the conversation. They are important because they let your student know that you are serious about finding out about his learning style. You want him to succeed, and you will help him to do so. As you begin work, and especially if problems appear, plan time for more conversation.

USE MULTISENSORY TEACHING METHODS

As much as is possible, find out about your student's particular learning style. Can he sit still and attend to lectures? Does he remember material presented auditorily, or does he gain more from print? Some of this information can be obtained by your initial conference with the student. If you can, also check records and ask other teachers about what types of teaching methods have been effective in the past.

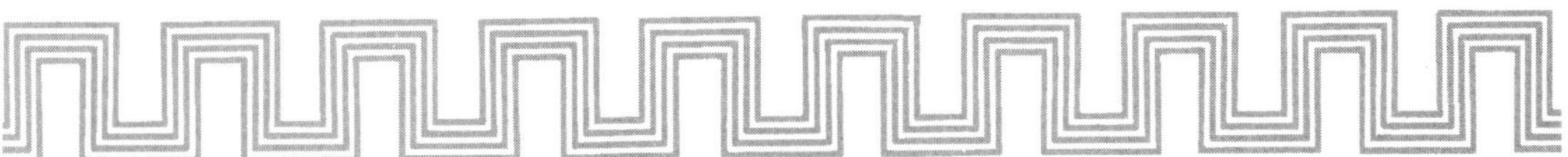

FINDING OUT ABOUT LEARNING STYLE

1. Which of the following helps you remember new information?

    reading about it ________

    hearing about it ________

    writing about it ________

2. Tell me more about this:

    ____

    ____

    ____

3. Does it help you to do a project using new information? ________ What are some projects that you have done that have helped you learn things?

    ____

    ____

    ____

4. Do you like to learn a series of facts first and then understand how they fit together, or do you like to have an overview first of how and why the facts are important?

    ____

    ____

5. (Present samples of books and/or other text media, including computer text, that you are planning on using.) How do you feel about reading things like this by yourself? Is the reading:

    very easy ________

    just about right ________

    okay, but it's hard because ____________________

    very difficult ________

Name ______________________________ **Date** ________________

FINDING OUT ABOUT LEARNING STYLE *(Cont'd)*

How do you feel about reading aloud a book like this?

____

____

____

6. Would you feel comfortable if I asked you to write:

    words __________

    sentences __________

    paragraphs __________

    reports __________

    How do you feel about your spelling and grammar?

    ____

    ____

    ____

7. Does it help you to sit in a certain part of the room when you are listening to the teacher?

    ____

8. Does it help you to sit in a certain part of the room when you are doing your own work or reading?

    ____

9. Do you want me to know anything special about the way you learn so that I can be a good teacher for you?

    ____

    ____

    ____

Name ______________________________ **Date** ________________

My Learning Style

1. I like to learn new things by:

   Reading __________

   Listening __________

   Writing __________

   Doing things __________

   Of all the things listed above, I learn best by:

   ____

   ____

2. I like to: (choose one)

   Learn a lot of facts before I know how they fit together _____

   Have an overview of the subject before I learn specific facts _____

3. In this class, I am concerned about:

   ____

   ____

4. I think that it would help me to learn a lot in this class if my teacher would:

   ____

   ____

   ____

   ____

Name ____________________________ **Date** ________________

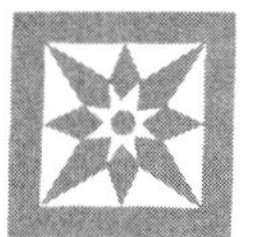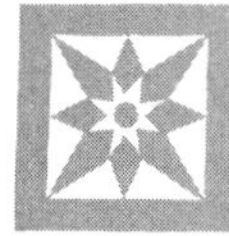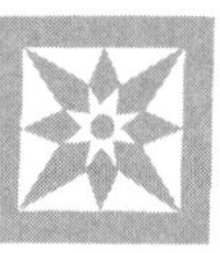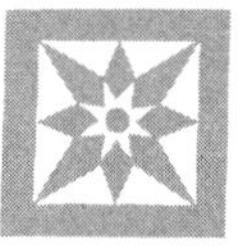

A Learning Contract

Date: ________________

As your teacher, I agree to do the following to help you learn:

____

____

____

If I have concerns, I will:

____

____

Signature of Teacher ______________________

As your student, I agree to do the following to help myself learn:

____

____

____

If I have concerns, I will:

____

____

Signature of Student ______________________

Name ______________________________ **Date** ________________

In general, the most effective teaching is varied. In presenting information, you want to have your students look and listen, to read about the information, and to write about it. You want them to discuss it—and most important, you want them to use the information and do something with it. Combine all of these modalities and you will have a very effective learning environment, not just for the student with dyslexia, but for all students.

Teach Students to Use Logic Rather than Rote Memory

For reading and spelling, students are taught the structure of the English language to help them remember details. For writing, math, and even handwriting, students discover concepts and utilize patterns to assist their rote memories. This same principle of grouping data into logical categories and groups will help in all subject areas. But how can a student with memory issues remember, for example, the bones of the body? At some point in academic life, students have to remember facts. For the student with dyslexia, keep in mind the following:

- Most students have a relatively stronger modality. For example, some will remember what they see better than what they hear, or vice versa. Some people will more easily remember data that they write down or use in different ways. The first job, therefore, is to find the strongest memory modality and then to help your student utilize this as the primary memorizing mode.

- The second important point is to limit the amount of specific data to be memorized to the absolute essential. Knowing huge numbers of facts can be helpful for succeeding in a television game show, such as *Jeopardy*, but it is not critically important for success in life.

- If students have difficulty with remembering a number of facts, it is important to have good research skills, so that they can quickly and easily find out what they want to know. For this reason, it is important to teach good library and computer skills. Teach students how to find out what they need to know. Inform them about the important resources in your field. Then, approach finding facts as a detective experience, posing questions to be answered and problems to be solved. Students will be interested and motivated to participate.

- For the facts that just have to be memorized, provide mnemonic devices. This helps because it adds meaning to relatively meaningless information. Some good mnemonic strategies are:

    1. Group data into groups of similar-sounding or looking words.

    2. Connect an unfamiliar new word with a known one. This works particularly well for people's first names. When a new person is introduced, invite students to mentally pair his name with either someone they already know with that name, or with a book character.

3. Create silly sentences, especially for things that must be remembered in sequence. For example, to memorize the order of the days of the week, you could help students create sentences like the following: "My teacher wants to find several spacecraft." The first letter of each word in the sentence is the same as the first letter in each day. Help students to make up their own sentences, and this will assist their memories.

4. Use visual aids and other tangible props that record the critical information. If students know that they can go back and check their memories, this will give them more confidence to really try to remember data.

PRESENT MATERIAL SEQUENTIALLY

This principle requires you to take an overview of the material you are presenting. This is true in art, music, and physical education, as well as in science and social studies. Look at your goals and your curriculum requirements for the year. For each unit, try to look at the most important elements. Then, present the less demanding and more accessible challenges first.

Experience building will provide your students with background information and interactions that will help them gain confidence. It will also provide a good backdrop for future learning. People remember best when facts and experiences are connected with one another.

Think of this sequential presentation of material as building a ladder. Once those early low rungs are strong, it is much easier to climb higher.

PRESENT MATERIAL IN SMALL UNITS

Teachers can feel overwhelmed by the amount of material they are expected to present. A common reaction is to "talk at" students, to give them large amounts of information verbally, so that the information is at least introduced in some way. Think for a moment, however, about how it feels to have someone "talk at" you in a monologue. Usually, in spite of your best efforts, your attention wanders, because it is difficult to maintain attention unless you are actively engaged.

Less is better. It's important to examine your curriculum for the essential elements. Break these into small units and present them thoroughly. This will not only create a positive learning environment for the student with dyslexia, but it will also be good for students with more traditional learning styles.

If you are asking your student to complete a written form or do some other written work that has several sections, it is most helpful to discuss one question or section at a time and then have the student complete that part. Then, go on to discuss the next section. This is a much better method than talking about everything in the beginning and then asking the student to complete the whole project at once. There is too much room for confusion with the excess of verbal directions in the latter approach.

For verbal directions in general, the basic principle is: Shorter is better. Here again, present information in small units. Some students with auditory memory issues have real difficulty with complex directions. In fact, it's a good idea to notice how many sequential directions, called "steps," your student can understand and remember. Some students can handle only one-step directions, like "Please take out your notebook," whereas others are able to respond to two-step directions, like "Please take out your notebook and open it up to the section on botany." Knowing how many sequential directions your students can understand and respond to effectively will make the learning environment much happier for everyone.

Practice, Practice, Practice, and Review

Students with dyslexia need a great deal of reinforcement when learning concepts and facts, but how can this be provided in the midst of a busy classroom?

First, try to isolate the essential information you want your student to learn. Then, try to provide extra experiences with this information using modalities other than just verbalization, especially modalities in which your student is strong.

Imagine, for example, that you have a student who is very talented in art. You are studying midwestern states and you want your student to remember a few state capitals and some important geographical information such as names of rivers. In this situation, you could invite your student to be in charge of a group project. He needs to plan out a large map that will be used as a paper mural. Once he has drawn the outlines of the states and placed their capitals and important geographical features, he can record the names. Then, he can invite his classmates to help him complete the map by coloring it and adding other graphics.

As the group is working, say things like "Who is going to color in the Colorado River?" If the information is used in meaningful contexts, it will be easier to remember.

Help Students Organize Time and Space

Organizational skills are a critical area of need for students with dyslexia. The following are some particular suggestions for dealing with organizational issues for related subjects.

Organizing Time. At the beginning of each class period, it is very helpful to tell students what the plan is for the day. Say approximately how much time will be allotted to each activity. This helps students know what they can expect in the time ahead. It also models for them how a large amount of time can be broken down into manageable units.

For short-term assignments, such as writing a summary of an experiment in science, discuss in advance how much time your student feels it will take him to complete the task. It can be particularly helpful to ask him to make and record an official estimate, and then to go back later to check how much time it actually took him. In this way, your student will learn to make realistic estimates of work time needed.

To help your students become highly reflective about how they use their time, ask them to keep an "Organizing My Time Journal." Here, they record thoughts and impressions about how they are managing with classroom assignments. This journal needs to be a very safe and supportive tool, in which students feel free to record their failures as well as their successes. One example of an "Organizing My Time Journal" is provided on page 215.

For long-term assignments, provide real structure and support. Assignments of this type are by their very nature difficult for students with dyslexia. Sit with your student and help him break the large task into the particular jobs that have to be done. Write each of these jobs on a piece of paper. For example, if your student is expected to write a report on World War II, you could list such things as the following:

- Research information by going to the library and finding at least three books that have information about the war.
- Talk to my grandfather who was a soldier in the war.
- Make preliminary notes about information to include.
- Make an outline.
- Write a first draft.
- Edit the first draft.
- Ask my older sister to edit the first draft.
- Make a final copy.

Once these jobs are listed, help your student make an estimate of how much time each one will take. Then, make a plan as to when he will work on each task. An independent activity sheet, "My Project," is provided on page 216 as an example of one way to structure this organizing effort.

Organizing Space. The classroom setting needs to be neat and uncluttered. Extraneous stimuli need to be removed as much as possible.

Physical organizers like large plastic bins or boxes should be utilized for storing objects not in use. As much as space permits, these organizers should be neatly arranged.

The student's work area needs to be neat and clutter free. The major stimuli present should deal with the concepts currently being studied.

Make sure that there are physical props for storing students' work. Three-ring binders with tabs for sectioning off work are particularly effective. It's recommended that students have a three-ring folder for each subject. These should be kept in the room so that loss of the folder is never an issue. Homework folders are maintained separately and will be discussed in the "Homework" section of this chapter.

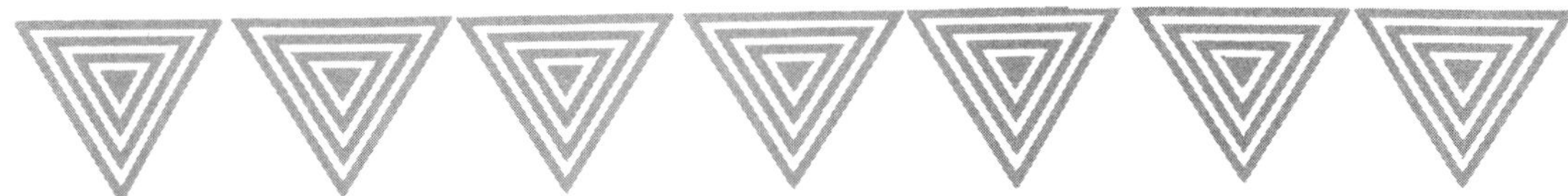

ORGANIZING MY TIME JOURNAL

Today, I was asked to do the following job in class:

____

I thought it would take me this many minutes: ________

It actually took me this many minutes: ________

It was (choose one):

Easy for me to start work ________

Difficult to start because ____________________________

It was (choose one):

Easy for me to keep working ________

Difficult to keep working because ______________________

I was (choose one):

Able to finish the project ________

Not able to finish the project ________

Today, in terms of organizing my time, I think I:

____

I think that it would help me to:

____

____

Name ____________________________ **Date** ________________

My Project

My project is:

____

What I have to do for this project | The time this will take

____

____

____

____

____

____

____

What I will do first, second, and so on | When I will start

1. ____

2. ____

3. ____

4. ____

5. ____

6. ____

7. ____

Name ______________________ **Date** ______________

Have consistent expectations for how students structure their written work. Each page should have

- a title
- the name of the student
- the date

It's also recommended that wide-lined, as opposed to college-lined paper be used, and that students skip lines. It's best to write on only one side of the paper, so that if changes in the organizational structure of the written product need to be made, students can easily cut and paste their writing onto a new sheet of paper.

Provide pencils and other necessary supplies. Students with dyslexia don't lose things because they want to; they do so because of innate organizational weakness. Creating a punitive environment for this weakness only makes students tense, and it does not help them at all. You can refer to Chapter 12, "Teaching Everyday Skills," for information on how to help students deal with their tendency to lose things.

Periodically, have a classroom clean-out time. Take an area of the classroom and model how to remove extraneous objects and how to organize what remains. Also periodically, have a student work area and notebook clean-out day. Help students decide what is essential and what needs to be thrown away. Model organizing the remaining objects and papers.

If you are giving out handouts or other papers, try to avoid visual clutter on the pages. The most effective handouts will be neat and organized, with limited visual stimuli.

When writing on the board or on a large paper, keep the text simple and keep the visual clutter to a minimum.

Individualize Instruction

This principle, on the surface, seems extremely difficult to accomplish. How can a busy teacher attend to the needs of one student, when there are so many others who also have needs?

Whereas it is true that every student in a classroom deserves careful attention, planning for the student with dyslexia often requires more conscious effort on the teacher's part. The standard curriculum has generally been designed with the traditional learner in mind and curriculum already meets his needs. Thus, it makes sense to spend some extra time planning for the learner with a nontraditional learning style.

What are some of the ways in which you can individualize instruction? First of all, you need to be aware of all the general principles, asking yourself the three basic questions:

1. Am I presenting information effectively to this student?
2. Is the student interacting well with the information?
3. Am I fairly assessing his knowledge?

Then, you can do things like the following:

For Question 1: Am I presenting information effectively to this student?

- Be very aware of whether or not the student is understanding your directions. Do you need to give directions with fewer steps?
- Present information utilizing talking, showing, and doing.
- Present information in a relatively distraction free environment.

For question 2: Is the student interacting well with the information?

- Make sure that your student can read all of the written directions.
- Ask yourself whether he has the basic reading and writing skills to complete projects and experiments. If not, either modify expectations or provide support.
- Ask yourself if he needs a different type of project. For example, instead of always having to complete a traditional written report, can he create and provide a skit for the class? Or can he make up a board game that utilizes information being studied?
- Provide a relatively distraction free environment in which he can work. A quiet corner can be such a space.

For Question 3: Am I fairly assessing his knowledge?

- Make sure that your student has the necessary basic skills of reading and writing to deal with written tests.
- Provide a relatively distraction-free environment.
- Notice if he has severe test taking anxiety that negatively affects his ability to perform.
- Ask yourself if he needs alternative types of assessment, such as oral tests or portfolio assessment.

The subject of assessment will be discussed in more detail later in this chapter.

In addition to individualizing for academic issues, it can also be important to individualize for behavior. Many students with dyslexia have ADD or ADHD. They can have impaired self-confidence and other emotional issues. Spend some time figuring out what they need, and provide some simple help like the following:

- A one minute check-in conversation every day to see how the student is feeling about his school performance.
- A contract system that holds both student and teacher accountable to agreed upon standards. A reproducible contract, "What I Will Do," is provided on page 219.

What I Will Do

Date: ____________________

As your teacher, I agree to do the following to help you be a conscientious and excellent student every day:

____

____

____

If you are experiencing difficulty during class, I will:

____

____

Signature of Teacher ___________________________

As your student, I agree to do the following to help me be a conscientious and excellent student every day:

____

____

____

If I am experiencing difficulty during class, I will:

____

____

Signature of Student ____________________

Name _____________________________________ **Date** ____________________

- A private and agreed-upon system, such as a gesture, for alerting the student to any of his inappropriate behavior. Dealing with behavior and with social and emotional needs will be discussed in detail in Chapters 15 and 16.

To summarize, it takes effort and time to individualize instruction for the student with dyslexia. It can take even more time, however, if you don't. How can you estimate what is lost in the classroom when a student is acting inappropriately? And if a student continues to fail with curriculum, look at the time lost for both the teacher and the student in dealing with this failure. Wouldn't you rather do some careful planning, and then be able to enjoy your student's success?

Always Be Aware of the Emotional Climate

Most students with dyslexia have experienced so much failure in the past that they can become highly insecure and nervous around any new academic challenge. This discomfort may arise unexpectedly. Your student may have been comfortably and successfully working for several weeks, and all of a sudden, he is becoming resistive. Why? Has your style of teaching changed? Have the expectations subtly changed? For example, are students volunteering to read aloud sections of interesting articles or texts, thus putting subtle pressure on your student to do the same? Or have you begun a new class project in which a different modality is being used? Are you, for example, studying the stages of early humanity, and are students being asked to create clay models of types of skulls? On the surface, this would seem to be a very appropriate activity: It's nonverbal, it utilizes three-dimensional, hands-on materials, and it's interactive. It's interesting and fun for most students. Your student with dyslexia, however, also experiences tactile defensiveness. Not much is known about this condition, but some people are overly stimulated by the sense of touch and are repelled by the feel of certain substances. Your student may be very disturbed by the feel of the clay, but he is too embarrassed to tell you or his peers about this. Therefore, he chooses to act uninterested in the activity and withdraws into silence.

The most important thing to do is to watch your student. If he is not functioning normally, set aside a private time and try to discover the cause so that the situation can be corrected.

Laugh a Lot

Again, this is so simple that it seems unnecessary to discuss. Teachers and students today, however, are under a great deal of pressure to "perform." The current emphasis on accountability and standardized testing makes everyone tense at some level. What are the best antidotes? Careful planning and laughter. Laughter will help everyone relax into the joy of learning.

RELATED SUBJECTS

In this section, we will briefly discuss the particular areas of social studies, science, art, music, and physical education, giving specific hints for effective lessons. These hints are not meant to be exhaustive. They are meant, instead, to give a general idea of the types of things that can be done to maximize learning for your student with dyslexia.

SOCIAL STUDIES

This area of learning is, at its essence, a study of the story of civilization. Students with dyslexia love stories. In addition, they enjoy discovering patterns and trends and overlying principles. They will respond to the challenge of figuring out why groups of people have reacted in the ways they have done in the past. They will enjoy trying to figure out what these people are likely to do in the future. Once they have done this type of study, they will be much more motivated to remember particular facts like people's names and the dates of important events.

Hints

- Approach the story of an important event, such as the Revolutionary War, by first presenting the story of an individual who lived at the time. Good historical fiction can be particularly helpful with this. For example, in the novel *Jordan Freeman Was My Friend* by Richard White (Four Walls Eight Windows, 1994), a boy named Billy tells the true story of the massacre of Americans by Benedict Arnold and his men in 1781. Rather than just a series of facts on a page, this book makes the story come alive through the eyes of a person.
- If studying a culture or an area of the world, read folk tales from those places. These tales can lead to good discussion about how these stories evolved, and how they themselves may have influenced the culture. A particularly good book for this purpose is *Thirty-Three Multicultural Tales to Tell* by Pleasant DeSpain, illustrated by Joe Shlichta (A Merrill Court Press Book published by August House Publishers, Inc., 1993). This book has great stories, and they are short, which makes it possible to read one a day as a part of the lesson.
- Use a lot of three-dimensional projects. Are you studying geography? Can your students, for example, make a topographical map of an area being studied? How about a mobile, in which students make a map of a place being studied on heavy paper, color it and cut it out, and then hang symbols of important geographical features from its base? The whole project can hang from a coat hanger attached to the ceiling.
- Don't forget about food. Are you studying China, for example? Try researching types of food from the different areas of China. Then, create a menu, a shopping

list, and a plan for preparation. Prepare one or two simple dishes and enjoy! Always be sure, when you are dealing with food, that you know of and do not use any food to which your students may be allergic.

- Diversify each lesson. Rather than having a whole hour's session of presenting information and then starting a project the next class day, discuss the topic for half the class and then get right on to that interactive project.

SCIENCE

Science is the discovery of important principles and facts that govern our physical world. This is an area with which many people with dyslexia are fascinated, especially because it fits their learning style. To be a scientist, you have to have a natural curiosity and a willingness to observe carefully with great focus. It particularly helps if you can look at a group of data with an open and imaginative mind. These are exactly the strengths that many people with dyslexia possess. Think of the famous scientist Michael Farraday, who made many important discoveries in chemistry and physics, and who is now believed to have had the learning style of dyslexia.

Hints

- Use three-dimensional, hands-on activities to introduce concepts. If you are studying levers, for example, have students first make a lever. Structure the lesson so that they discover that there are different types of levers. Then, have students record their observations utilizing, first pictures and then words at whatever level they are writing. Even if they are writing at the word writing level, they can label their illustrations of their projects.

- Have an ongoing project that encourages observation of the natural world. Record the outside temperature at a certain time every day, for example, and make a chart of these numbers. Or choose an object such as a tree or a pole in a playground or park, and daily observe what happens to its shadow. Make observational notes about this. These types of activities are good for many reasons: They trigger interest about the natural world, they help develop observational skills, and they provide legitimate outlets for excess energy. If, for example, you have a student with ADHD who seems to be having particular difficulty with his hyperactivity on a given day, he can be the one you ask to go out and check the thermometer.

- Plant flowers or vegetables. If you're lucky enough to have an outside area for a garden, plan it, plant it, and enjoy the results. In colder climates, it works well to plant spring greens and edible pea pods in early spring because they'll be ready to harvest before school gets out. You can also plant squash and pumpkins, which will grow through the summer and be ready in the fall.

- It's helpful to have ongoing projects that engage varied modalities. Thus, in a given lesson, there can be great diversity that helps the student with dyslexia fully attend for the whole time.

- Listen to your students and allow creativity. Whereas it is important that students learn how to complete class assignments, they sometimes can get ideas that fascinate them and that they wish to pursue. Perhaps, for example, there is a box of old brass, copper, and other small metal objects in a junk box in the room. Your student decides that he wants to put them together so that he can make an invention. He doesn't yet know what he wants to make, but he clearly wants to experiment. Form a plan with this student, so that he is clear that he is still expected to participate in the regular class work. Also, however, plan for some time when he will be allowed to work on his independent project. It can be particularly effective to help him structure his experimentation; for example, this is one possible structure: He will freely explore the objects for a certain amount of time, decide upon what he wishes to accomplish, record this in some way either pictorially or in writing, and then proceed to create his invention. This helps the student realize that the scientific principles and procedures that he has been learning can be applied to his own creative experiments.

ART

So many students with dyslexia have real talent in this area, and yet others who have visual-motor difficulties do not enjoy the activity. Also, the field of art encompasses many skills and abilities. Some students will easily succeed in one area—three-dimensional work, for example—but will struggle with another, such as two-dimensional drawing.

Hints

- Even in this less formal academic area, lessons need to be structured. It helps to tell students what you are going to do for the day, where they will work, the materials they will use, and how much time will be needed for cleanup.
- Pay particular attention to the times of transition, so that students know what your expectations are for appropriate behavior. If you are aware that a student has difficulty during unstructured times, make a behavioral plan with him in advance.
- If a student is experiencing difficulty with a given project, notice the particular skills that are required and try to present activities that require different skills in the future. For example, on a given task, a lot of fine cutting with scissors is required. Your student is having great difficulty handling the scissors and getting them to cut properly. You have noticed in the past, however, that he happily spent hours constructing a three-dimensional model home out of boxes, cardboard, and other findings. Provide projects that allow him to work in his area of strength and interest. If you wish to help him improve his cutting skills, address these at a separate time. It can be particularly helpful in a case like this to consult an occupational therapist so that you can learn the prerequisite skills for effectively using scissors.

- Some students have tactile defensiveness, or the aversion to touching or being touched. With some students, the symptoms can be more severe with particular textures, such as papier-mâché or clay. Tactile defensiveness is a real problem for some students, and it is not something that they would choose to experience. They therefore need understanding and support. Discuss their difficulties privately, and make a plan for coping with them.

MUSIC

This is another area in which students with dyslexia can flourish, and, in fact, there are many stories about people who either sing beautifully or who easily learn musical instruments. But as we have seen over and over, students with dyslexia are extremely diverse in their surprising strengths and weaknesses. Therefore, you have to watch each student carefully.

Hints

- As with all subjects, it helps to tell students what is going to happen in a given class time. Will you learn a new song and then practice some old ones? Will homemade rhythm instruments be created and used? Knowing what is going to happen can help students feel safe.
- Be particularly careful about transitions, those times, for example, when musical instruments or sheet music are being gathered or put away. For students with ADHD, these times can be full of pitfalls. They can start playing with the instruments, or making paper airplanes out of the sheet music. Help to avoid this behavior by structuring all aspects of the class. Perhaps one student can get the music while others wait and sing a song.
- Another important consideration is to make sure that difficulties with academics do not interfere with the enjoyment of the music. Ask yourself questions like "Can my student read the words on the sheet music?" "Do his eyes jump around a page, rather than traveling from left to right and then easily down to the next line?" This eye-tracking issue can affect reading musical notations as well as words. "Am I expecting too much memory work if I am asking my students to memorize several songs?"
- Remember that music can be very supportive to the acquisition of academic skills. For example, a father of a student once reported that he didn't learn to read as a child. Throughout his school career, he stumbled and struggled with words. As an adult, however, he started attending church and began to sing along with the congregation as they sang hymns. Week after week, he experienced the connection between the words on the hymnal pages and the words he was hearing and singing. This taught him how to read. Now, he reads with fluency and enjoyment.

Physical Education

Some students with dyslexia are talented athletes. They can be stars on the football or basketball team, and this can be excellent for gaining self-esteem. Other have gross motor difficulties that inhibit their functioning with sports and other physical education activities. Balance, directionality, and motor coordination can be impaired.

Hints

- It helps to tell students what will happen during a class time.
- Vary games and activities within a class period so that different skills and abilities will be required.
- Make sure your directions for games and other activities are simple, with only one, two, or at the most, three steps at a time. For students with auditory memory issues, it doesn't help to repeat complicated directions, because they won't remember them any better the second or even the third time. They need directions that are simple and sequential.
- Carefully watch your students. Avoid activities and games that will embarrass them. If the class is participating in a game that you know is difficult for a student, see if you can set up an alternative activity.
- Cooperative games, in which competition is not a factor, are good choices for students who are insecure with their physical abilities.
- Physical education teachers have a unique opportunity to observe the student who is experiencing balance or directionality or other issues. Sometimes, a student needs remedial training from an occupational or physical therapist, and if this is provided in a timely way, it can greatly help him in all phases of his school life. If you feel that a student may need this type of help, talk with your school psychologist and/or special education teacher. They may wish to come and observe the student. Don't be reluctant to seek this type of help. If in doubt, err on the side of overreferring.

HOMEWORK

There are few other areas that can create such hardship and frustration as homework. If properly structured, however, homework can be empowering. It can be something that makes a student feel, "I can do that. I'm good." Homework is also a fact of life for all levels of schoolwork, so it's very important to establish good habits right from the beginning.

Some basic principles are:

- Homework should be a practice experience, in which concepts that have been studied and mastered are utilized. Homework should never be a vehicle for presenting new information.

- Keep directions simple. One-, two-, or at the most, three-step directions are best.
- The amount of homework should be reasonable. It's helpful to check with parents and other guardians to see how much time students are spending. If they are unable to complete the homework in a mutually agreed upon reasonable amount of time, the homework amount should be modified. Generally, people agree that elementary school students should spend approximately one hour a day on homework, whereas secondary students should spend approximately two hours.
- The difficulty level of the homework should be such that students can complete it independently. It does nothing for a student's self esteem or for his learning if he is constantly needing assistance in order to complete an assignment.
- Students usually need help in planning their homework time, and in figuring out how they are going to prioritize and approach tasks, especially if they have multiple assignments or assignments with multiple steps. Some of these helps are:
    1. A homework folder or notebook, in which all sheets that need to be taken home are placed. Provide a good amount of support in placing these sheets at first. Keep as your goal, however, that the student will become more independent with this.
    2. A homework log, in which jobs for each day are listed. A two-page reproducible, "My Homework for Today," provides an example of one such homework log on pages 227 and 228. This includes a materials checklist, where all necessary books and other supplies are listed.
- Praise good effort. Even if the homework is not perfect, praise whatever genuine accomplishments are there.

ASSESSMENT

Everyone agrees that a student's progress needs to be tested. The amount of knowledge that he has mastered gives important clues for future programming. Students with dyslexia, however, often have serious issues with traditional testing, so much so that the test does not assess their true mastery of the subject. Some of these issues are:

- The actual reading of the text can be laborious and not fluent. Thus, the student has to concentrate on reading the questions, instead of being able to think of the right answer. This labored reading can be caused by:
    1. Limited reading skills, which make the decoding of the words difficult
    2. Eye-tracking problems, which make the reading slow and scattered
    3. Reading comprehension problems, which make understanding the questions hard

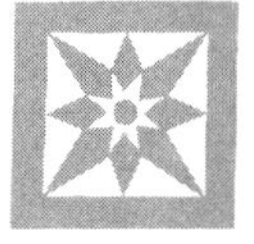 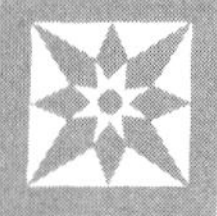 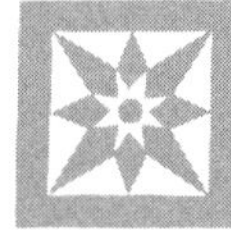  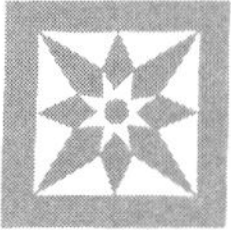  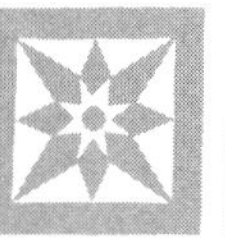  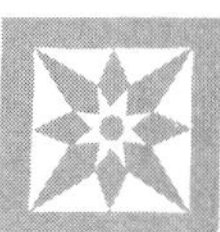

MY HOMEWORK FOR TODAY

These are the jobs that I have to do today:

	SUBJECT	WHAT I HAVE TO DO
1.	____________	______________________________
2.	____________	______________________________
3.	____________	______________________________
4.	____________	______________________________
5.	____________	______________________________

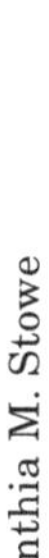

This is the order in which I will do my homework:

	JOB	HOW MUCH TIME IT WILL TAKE
1.	____________________	____________
2.	____________________	____________
3.	____________________	____________
4.	____________________	____________
5.	____________________	____________

If I have a long project due for (subject) ______________________
on (date) ____________, I will do the following for that project:

____

____

____

____

Name ________________________ **Date** ______________

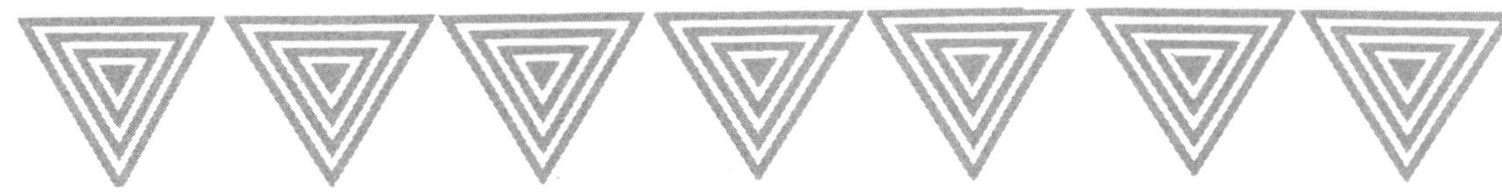

My Homework for Today *(Cont'd)*

These are the materials I will need:

SUBJECT	BOOKS	NOTEBOOK	PENCIL	OTHER
______________	______________	_____	_____	______________
______________	______________	_____	_____	______________
______________	______________	_____	_____	______________
______________	______________	_____	_____	______________
______________	______________	_____	_____	______________
______________	______________	_____	_____	______________

To help myself do a good job on my homework, this is the place I will work:

____

____

To help myself have lots of energy for my homework, this is the time of day I will work: ____

____

To help myself not be distracted, I will: ________________________________

____

Name ________________________________ **Date** __________________

- Syntax issues can confuse students, especially on multiple-choice tests. Here, the student can get confused by the order of the words and wonder what the question is really asking.
- Writing the answers can be hard. If students are not yet fluent writers, they may know the answer but may not be able to easily express this in words.
- Penmanship issues, either with speed or legibility, can limit a student's presentation of information.
- A great deal of visual stimuli on a test page can distract and confuse the student. He can spend too much time focusing on the extraneous stimuli, rather than on the important questions.
- A limited ability to focus on and attend to a two-dimensional task can hamper his performance.

The following recommendations help to make sure that assessment is fair:

- Provide a distraction-free test-taking environment.
- Consider portfolio assessment. Here, samples of a student's work are dated and saved in an orderly fashion. One can examine the work to see how he is progressing.
- If traditional multiple choice or essay tests are required, give students with dyslexia an unlimited amount of time. This helps compensate for the reading speed issue, and also helps the student relax so that he can really demonstrate his knowledge.
- If a student is a beginning reader or writer, give an oral test.
- Modify the test structure to realistically take into account the reading and writing levels, penmanship, and other spatial abilities.
- Consider alternative forms of assessment, such as projects, presentations, and reports. Through them, a student can truly demonstrate what he knows.

A SUMMARY

Students with dyslexia can succeed with all the challenges inherent in related subjects. Form a learning team with your student and then enjoy his successes.

Do expect

- good effort
- care with every project and paper

- honesty regarding how difficult or easy a task or activity really is
- a request for help when the work or activity seems too difficult

Don't expect:

- perfect spelling
- perfect grammar
- a completely neat product with no spatial issues
- the same level of performance every day. Because dyslexia is a neurological condition, it can affect students more on some days than on others. That is why many teachers become discouraged. They say, "He could do it yesterday." Expect this variation in performance. It's not based on motivation or behavior; it's truly part of the learning style. To help your student with this variation in performance ability, notice carefully what he can do each day, and try to adjust your presentation of information and expectations for that day only.

INTERVIEW WITH DANIEL

Daniel, a 15-year-old student at a small school for students with special needs, talks about types of instruction.

Let's talk about social studies and science.

Well, I don't really like either of them. I like when we go outside and do gardening and stuff like that, but they do too much talking. We need to do more stuff. They talk too much. The teacher talks too much. But I liked it when Ms. Chen was here. We colored in maps and put little points on where things are.

What are you studying right now in social studies?

We're studying early humans, like the different kinds like Homo Sapiens—stuff like that. We're studying about skulls. And in science we're studying about rocks. Rocks are pretty fun, because you get to look at the rock and identify what it is. That's pretty fun. We look at it through a telescope, not a telescope, a . . . whatever that thing is that makes it bigger. What is that? I forget what it's called.

A microscope?

Yeah. A microscope. I like social studies. I like coloring maps and identifying where things are and stuff like that. And it was fun when we went to the museum and I looked at a picture and I drew it, like the skull of a lizard, or something like that. I forget what it was. It was some sort of dinosaur, I think. And we wrote about it.

I'm hearing that you enjoy social studies and science when you're actually doing something, when you've got a project.

Yeah.

But you don't really like it when you're sitting and talking about it.

Right. What's the point? It's better to do something about it. And I like to do reports.

CHAPTER 12

TEACHING EVERYDAY SKILLS

It is in everyday life that dyslexia often surprises people, because this is where stark contradictions in ability become apparent. Why, for example, can't the bright 12-year-old girl with the active intellect and lively imagination simply not remember the days of the week? Why are the months of the year completely beyond her? And why, when you ask her what month comes next after February, will she sit and stare hopelessly at you?

Everyday life is often the place where the student with dyslexia can experience the most poignant incidents of embarrassment. Remember a phone number—her own, perhaps? This is sometimes impossible. When she is in school, she may be in a nurturing and supportive environment. Out there in the world, however, she will encounter many people who have little or no understanding of her struggles.

In this chapter, we will deal with six main areas: time, money, remembering important details, dealing with environmental print, keeping track of possessions, and a few specific problem areas. As we look at each of these areas, we must examine whether we can in fact teach the student with dyslexia how to overcome difficulties in these areas, or whether it is more prudent to develop creative compensations and to teach the student how to cope. In some cases, both approaches will be necessary.

TIME

Sometimes, this area is included in a math curriculum, in which students are taught how to tell time on a clock face. In this resource, however, it's included here, because many students with dyslexia have multiple and ongoing issues with many aspects of time. When they are children, this difficulty can make them fail to meet the expectations of parents and teachers, and thus, they are always "in trouble." When they are adults, it can be a serious impediment to positive social relationships and success on the job. They can have difficulty with the following:

- Telling time
- The language of time
- How to be "on time"
- How not to waste time

We will discuss each of these areas, in turn.

TELLING TIME

Most students with dyslexia have significant difficulty learning how to tell time. They often do not understand what the numbers on the clock face mean. Rarely are they able to glance at a conventional circle clock and say the time. If proper instruction is provided, however, they can adequately learn this important skill.

When you teach how to tell time, the following are extremely important:

1. Check that your students have an understanding of number concepts. These should include one to twelve for the hours, and one to sixty for the minutes. Don't assume that they know what the numerals represent. They may have been hiding a lack of understanding for years.
2. Teach that there are sixty minutes in every hour.
3. Become aware of the odd language used in telling time. As adults who have been telling time for years, we automatically say, "It's ten to one." "It's a quarter of three." "It's half past seven." What does that mean to a person not familiar with the expressions? What do "ten to" and "a quarter of" and "half past" mean? Once you become aware of the difficult expressions involved in telling time, you will be much more able to point them out and work with them.
4. Use old clock faces, or make your own with cardboard. Students need to feel the clock face and the two hands, as they move the hands and say the times represented. Multisensory instruction is very important here.
5. Teach that there are two hands on the clock face, and that one represents the hours and the other represents the minutes. Some teachers prefer to make up their own clock faces, so that they can provide different colors for the two hands. You can also create a different texture for the minute hand; for example, you can cover it with glue and then sprinkle fine sand on it.
6. On a clock face, show your students how the hour hand changes once the minute hand has gone fully around the circle. Have students do this many times.
7. Show students that there are two number systems on the clock face, and explain to them that this is why telling time is so difficult. The numbers printed on most clock faces are the hours: one, two, three, and so forth. The minute hand, however, moves around using a different system. When the minute hand reaches the

"one," we say that it has gone five minutes. Usually, it is best to introduce this confusing aspect by grouping the minutes into fives, and then helping students learn to count them by saying what each hour number means for the minutes. Then, you can start looking at the numbers in between. There is no fast way to do this, but practicing with three-dimensional clocks and clock hands does eventually work. You just have to make everything explicit.

8. Games also help, because they provide practice and a real purpose for telling time. One such game utilizes a set of dice and a clock face that is set to twelve o'clock for each student. In turn, students roll the dice and add up the number. This is the number of minutes they can move the minute hand. They then do this and say the time on their own clocks, which they have thus created. The winner is the person who has gotten to the latest "time" at the end of the game.

Some people suggest that students with dyslexia simply be given a digital clock. Why spend so much instructional time on a skill that is not absolutely essential because there is another device that can be used?

First, even when students read off the numbers on a digital clock, as in "It's 12:35," they can be confused about what the numbers mean without proper instruction. In addition, not being able to read a conventional clock can embarrass them when this skill is required in social situations.

The Language of Time

As with telling time, it's important to assess whether your student has an understanding of the general terms associated with time. Does she, for example, know the difference between "yesterday" and "tomorrow?" Are the terms "past," "present," and "future" truly clear? How about "sooner" and "later?" These abstract terms can be awkward both to understand and to use in conversational speech. Thus, it is very helpful to be aware of the particular language terms that pose difficulties, and to provide direct instruction for them.

How to Be "On Time"

People with traditional learning styles generally have an innate sense of time. Even if such a person has no access to a clock for a few hours, she has a sense of about what time it is. Many people with dyslexia do not have this ability. Hours can go by, and they are not completely aware of it.

This can cause great stress. Children don't come home when they're supposed to. Adults are so late for appointments that the other person has left. It is a common trait for the person with dyslexia not to be "on the same clock" as her peers. She is often judged to be irresponsible because of this behavior.

Most people agree that, in this area, coping skills need to be taught. Sometimes, for example, it is suggested that children tell responsible adults when they are supposed to go somewhere, and ask them to signal them when it is time to leave. Another suggestion is to have an alarm set on a digital watch that will alert the person to a time limit. A third is to combine some environmental stimulus with a time. For example, a teacher could say, "Come back from the library when the first graders go past to go to lunch."

Each case is different, and it's very important to discuss the issue directly with your student and to make a plan. She may be able to invent good clues for herself, which will alert her to a time deadline. The plan you make together may have to be modified, but eventually, something that will help alleviate the problem will be created.

How Not to Waste Time

Students with dyslexia can have a different sense of how time passes. They don't, for example, always experience the extreme differences between the passage of a few minutes and an hour. Some people believe that this is because of the intense concentration that they can have, which "turns off" the inner time sense. Whether they are tying a shoe or setting the table or pursuing an academic interest, they are focusing only on the job, not on the time passing.

You can teach strategies to help. See Chapter 11 for the "Organizing My Time Journal" and other strategies. You can also teach coping strategies. As with the issues involved with being "on time," discuss the need to be occasionally focused on other people's schedules. For example, they may need to dress quickly in the morning so that they can catch the school bus. If they really can only dawdle in the morning, then, they need to get up earlier. They may need to move along on that research project so that they can finish a report when it is due. Talking about these issues helps, and often it is the student herself who can come up with effective coping strategies.

MONEY

Although almost all students with dyslexia have some issues with time, only some have difficulties with money. We will discuss two main areas that pose particular challenges: counting money and using banks, such as with checkbooks.

Counting Money

There is a wonderful poem called *Smart*! in *Where the Sidewalk Ends: Poems and Drawings* by Shel Silverstein (HarperCollins, 1974). In this poem, the speaker tells about how smart he is because he was able to trade two quarters for one dollar, and everybody knows that two is a higher number than one. The speaker is right—it is confusing. How can one nickel be worth the same as five pennies? And that dime is a lot smaller than the nickel but it's worth twice as much?

When teaching about money, it's important to do the following:

1. Assess your students' knowledge of number concepts. If they are not secure in their understanding, wait to introduce work with money until they are. It will only confuse them to add another element to that initial work.

2. Check that they understand what the various forms of money represent. Dollars are generally easier than pennies, nickels, dimes, and quarters. Don't just ask them what they know, but instead create situations in which they have to show you. This should be done in a safe and private environment, so that if they don't know some basic facts, they won't be embarrassed in front of their peers.

3. Once you clearly know what your students need to work with, use money to teach money. Some teachers use actual coins, whereas others feel more comfortable with play money. The latter should be close in form to real money.

4. Use a lot of props, multisensory reinforcing stimuli. For example, make sure that there is a chart or a poster on which it is represented that five pennies are equal in value to one nickel, that five nickels are equal in value to one quarter, and that four quarters are equal in value to one dollar. Have these props prominently displayed so that students can readily refer to them.

5. Provide many opportunities for students to handle and work with the money. Some things to do are:

   - Show students two small piles of coins (the number of coins in each pile is determined by the students' level), and ask them to tell you which pile represents the most money.
   - Show your students some coins and ask them to figure out their value.
   - Ask your students to exchange money; for example, show them a dime and a quarter, and ask them to represent that same amount of money using different coins.
   - Have a small "store," where either pictures of things or small objects are arranged. Every object has a price, from one penny to a dollar, written on it. Tell your students that you are going to practice counting money and making change. Tell them right at the beginning that this is for practice and that they will not be able actually to purchase the items. If you are working with a small group, have students take turns being the storekeeper. Every student is given the same amount of money to "spend," and they take turns doing so. If change is required, the storekeeper counts out the appropriate amount from the store's cash register. Even older students enjoy working with the store, and it helps them become comfortable with money, even with making change.

USING BANKS

With just a little attention, students can become comfortable with banking. The first thing you need to assess is their ability to deal with banking forms, especially checks, deposit slips, and withdrawal slips. Simplified versions of these forms, "Checks" and "Banking Forms" (from *Let's Write!* by Cynthia M. Stowe, The Center for Applied Research in Education, 1997), are provided on pages 239 and 240. Your students can use them for practice.

If you ask, parents and other teachers often have outdated accounts with extra blank checks. If you carefully cross out names to emphasize that these checks are being used for practice, you can gain some good, authentic materials to use.

The Eagle Mountain School in Greenfield, Massachusetts, has an excellent program for teaching banking skills. Students are paid a salary in Eagle Mountain dollars (pretend money) at the end of each month. They can also earn Eagle Mountain dollars by doing extra work and winning games. They write checks when expenses occur, such as purchasing an item from a catalogue that is provided. Once the check is written, they have to keep an account of the money left. Even though all the money and purchases are for practice only and are not real, students still greatly enjoy practicing with money in this way.

REMEMBERING IMPORTANT DETAILS

Part of the dyslexic learning style can be an inherent weakness in the following two areas: (1) rote auditory memory, especially of language that has little inherent meaning, and (2) sequencing skills.

These two weaknesses can make learning such things as the days of the week, the months of the year, and phone numbers very difficult. And these are important, because while they are not inherently critical for success at school or on the job, people in our culture expect others to be fluent with them. People who do not know something that "everybody" knows are judged to be inferior.

Fortunately, direct instruction can help. In terms of the names of the days and months, it is best to start with the days, because these are easier. You can approach this in the following way:

1. Clearly associate each day with an event, as much as is possible. For example, "Monday is usually the first day of school. Tuesday, we have art in the afternoon." This list of associations can be different for each student.
2. Another helpful thing is to talk about the history of the name of each day. These can be found in any good etymology book.
3. Once students are familiar with the names, start working on the sequence. Work with questions like "What day comes after Thursday? What day comes before Sunday?"

CHECK

Date ____________________ 20 _____

Pay to the
order of ____ $_______

____ Dollars

(write in words)

____
Signature

CHECK

Date ____________________ 20 _____

Pay to the
order of ____ $_______

____ Dollars

(write in words)

____
Signature

Name ________________________________ **Date** ____________________

DEPOSIT SLIP

Name ______________________

Addresss ______________________

____

Date ______________________

Account # ______________________

Cash		
Checks		
Total		

WITHDRAWAL SLIP

Date ______________________

Pay to me or ______________________

Amount of money __________ ______________________

(write in words)

Signature ______________________

Address ______________________

Account # ______________________

Name ______________________ **Date** ______________________

4. Help students learn to say the names in sequence. Here, a mnemonic device is often helpful; they remember a seven word sentence in which each word starts with the first letter of the day of the week, in order. One such sentence is "My teacher wants to find several spaceships."

5. As you go through these stages of teaching the days of the week, provide written models. Also, multisensory projects can be helpful. For example, students can make a poster of all the things that they like to do on a Saturday.

Unless your students are very advanced in spelling, don't expect them to be able to spell the names correctly without a prop. Your initial goal is for them to know the names of the days and to be able to talk about them easily in school and social contexts.

Teaching the months of the year follows the same steps as the days of the week. It is somewhat easier to create a common association with each month; for example, "Valentine's Day is celebrated in February." Using a mnemonic device for remembering the sequence, however, is more difficult, because a twelve-word sentence is just too much to remember.

The third area of important details to remember is phone numbers. Here, it is usually best to develop coping strategies, as remembering series of numbers that have relatively little meaning is a common and serious difficulty. Talk with your student about how many phone numbers she wishes to remember. Can she remember her own phone number rather easily? If she cannot, can she think of a way to carry this with her? Does she need to remember her mother's phone number at work? Does she want to carry a little notebook in which she can record important numbers? How about a hand-held computer device? It is important to help your student create her own system, so that when she is on her own, she will be able to adapt successfully to meet new demands. One specific hint you can give your student is to tell her that it is acceptable to ask people to repeat a number that they have given you. Teach her to say something like "Will you repeat that number, please, while I write it down?"

DEALING WITH ENVIRONMENTAL PRINT

There are written words and numbers everywhere in our culture. Some important examples are

- Calendars
- Catalogues
- Menus
- Bus and train schedules
- Job applications
- Newspapers
- TV guides

The following help students become comfortable with these:

- Get actual samples of all of these types of products. You can get some of them from parents and peers. For others, such as menus, you can ask businesses to provide a sample. Businesses are usually very gracious once you explain what you are using their product for.
- With your students, examine the structure of each type of product. Take apart the newspaper, for example, and look at each section. Talk about where you can find different kinds of information.
- Use the product. For a practice experience with a menu, for example, tell students that they have a certain amount of pretend money with which to buy lunch. Ask them to use the menu to figure out what they will buy. They will have to figure out not only the total amount of the food cost, but also the tax and tip (great math practice). For practice filling out job applications, the reproducible "A Job Application" (from *Let's Write!*) is provided on page 243. This is a simplified version, and it is a good place to start learning how to fill out these critically important forms.
- Create a sample product. Have your students make a calendar for the classroom, or write out a menu for the school cafeteria.

All of the above, done at the level at which your students are functioning successfully, will help them relax outside of school. They will feel more prepared to face the demands of social situations.

KEEPING TRACK OF THINGS

A common trait of students with dyslexia is to lose things. They lose notebooks carrying them from one room to another. Pencils are misplaced almost before they are used. Some women don't carry purses because they are afraid they will lose them.

Sit with your student and define the problem. Talk about what you see happening, and elicit her feelings about her difficulty with keeping track of things. Is she upset about it? Does she want to try to develop coping strategies?

Finding out your student's feeling is the first thing to do, because if she is not uncomfortable with losing things, she will not be motivated to expend the great amount of energy required to change. Most students will express discomfort. If someone does not, tell her what you are observing in a nonjudgmental way; for example, "I noticed that yesterday, you didn't bring a pencil to class and you lost your sweater out at recess." Tell her that if she decides that she wants to do something about this in the future, she should tell you, and you will be glad to help her.

 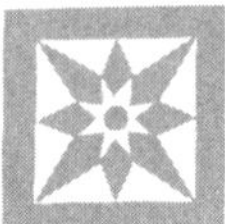 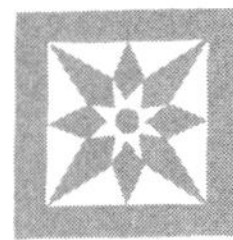 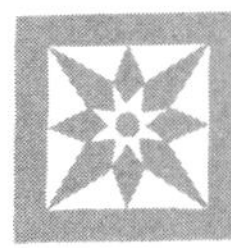  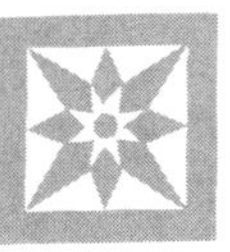 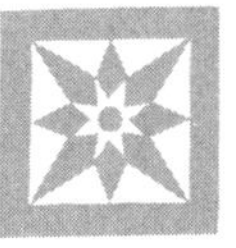 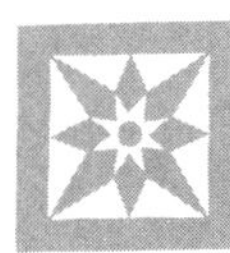 

A Job Application

Date ____________________

Name ____

Social security number ____________________

Address ____

Telephone number ____________________

Are you legally available for work in the U.S.A.? Yes _____ No _____

Name of your school ____

School address ____

Last grade completed ____

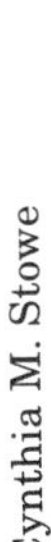

Employment Record

Company name ____

Address ____

Your position and duties ____

____

Why did you leave? ____

____

References

Name ______________________________ Phone ______________

Name ______________________________ Phone ______________

What kind of job are you seeking? ______________________________

Full or part time ______________

If your student expresses a desire to create some coping strategies, tell her that the following are helpful:

- creating specific places where things are routinely kept
- building good habits

Choose one object with which she would like to work. Is she tired, for example, of losing her homework notebook? She does have to bring this to school every morning and then back home at night. Ask your student to close her eyes and to envision what she does with her homework notebook when she walks in the door at home. Does she just throw it in her room on the floor? Does she not know what she usually does with it? Ask her to close her eyes again and to decide upon a place where she is going to place her notebook when she goes home that afternoon. Follow the same procedure for what she will do with it when she brings the notebook back to school.

Follow your student's progress with this one item. You can even make a chart of her successes with her new system. It's very important to celebrate her successes. If she fails, say something like "This is very hard for you, and you're not going to be able to do this perfectly right away. Don't worry. Remember that last week, you kept good track of your notebook for three days in a row. That's good progress. We'll just keep working on it."

Once your student has become very successful with one object, add another. But keep asking her how much effort she wants to expend. She may need periods of rest between focused times of work in this area.

A FEW SPECIFIC PROBLEM AREAS

The following specific areas can create great embarrassment for people with dyslexia. We will list a few first and then make suggestions for how your student can cope with them.

- ***Parties.*** There can be so many expectations when a large group of people get together. At one party, for example, guests were gathered around watching the birthday person opening her gifts. When it came time for one gift, the giver said, "Oh, read my card first. Read it out loud. It's really funny." The birthday person has great difficulty reading aloud, but how does she explain this when facing this large group?
- ***Games.*** So many games have so much text. The obvious ones like Scrabble™ are clearly dependent upon spelling and vocabulary. But what about Charades, in which a person must read a card in order to know what to act out? Many games require good ability with reading, spelling, and math.

- ***Art and Craft Projects or Puzzles.*** Some students with visual-motor difficulties become very nervous when they are asked to "perform" in this area in front of others. What if their club or church group, for example, is making some craft project for sale for fund raising? This can be a highly uncomfortable situation.
- ***Introducing People.*** Remembering people's names is difficult for many people, but especially so for the person with dyslexia. She can have difficulty with remembering the name and, sometimes, with pronouncing it.

The following suggestions help students cope with these everyday life challenges:

- For remembering names, a mnemonic strategy is recommended. Ask your student to try to associate a new person's name with either a friend or another familiar person with that same name. The trick is to add meaning to the unfamiliar name.
- Invite your student to be honest with someone about her difficulties with art projects and with games. Suggest that she choose a person who feels trustworthy, and then tell that person what makes her uncomfortable. If the social group has a leader, such as in a Girl Scout troop, this person can help her avoid potentially embarrassing situations.
- Discuss with your student what she feels comfortable telling people about her dyslexia in various social situations. If she has decided in advance what she feels comfortable saying to distant family members, social acquaintances, and strangers, this will help her deal with unexpected challenges.
- Help your student develop a list of games and other activities that she is comfortable with and that she can suggest at parties or at game times. Most often, everyone will be just as happy with her choices and will not even notice that she was reluctant to play another game.

INTERVIEW WITH NAOMI

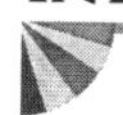

Here, Naomi, who was first interviewed in Chapter 2, speaks about how her son Malcolm has learned some skills that are essential for everyday life.

Was it hard for Malcolm to learn to tell time?

Uh huh. We actually went and . . . I went and bought one of these special clock things. You know, it has this thing that first you do it by hours and then you do it by half-hours and quarter-hours.

So you got a special clock?

Yes, and we used that at home as a game. The thing is that in school, they had digital clocks. I thought that was, really, not helpful.

What about counting change and dealing with money? Was that natural for Malcolm?

He did better with that.

So telling time was the issue.

Yeah. Malcolm has an entrepreneurial spirit. So that was a great motivation to learn how to count money. He used to set up tag sales at the end of our driveway, a running tag sale. When he got tired of his toys, he would take them down to the end of our driveway and sell things. He's creative around business things, he has lots of business ideas, ways to make money. Another thing is, he would take his Halloween candy to school and sell it to his friends. He wasn't big on candy. So he has an entrepreneurial spirit, so counting change came a little quicker.

So perhaps if time had been connected with something of high motivational value . . .

Yeah, it would have been easier.

And you said that Malcolm also has issues around organization.

Yes.

What about organizing time? How's that?

It was really an issue before. He's doing so much better now. Now he can figure out what to do with his time, like doing his homework and stuff like that. He's doing much better. He's also gotten into organizing his own desk, and we have different shelves, and he's got his computer stuff more organized.

But he's got an added challenge, because he's got to go between two houses. Most of the time he remembers. He's got his retainer to remember and his homework, and I think the hardest thing is sports equipment. You've got to think about what you're going to be doing at the end of the day or the next day. But I think he's come a long way with organizational things.

And that's come by working at it?

Yeah, I think so. I really think the method at school has really helped. That was one thing in his old school that hurt. They were moving more toward the open classroom. There was too much stimulus, too many choices, too much shifting from one thing to another. All of that kind of stuff was not supportive. I think it's great for some kids. It just doesn't work for Malcolm.

CHAPTER 13

ISSUES RELATED TO DYSLEXIA

In this chapter, we will briefly discuss three areas in which people with dyslexia can have difficulties. These are

- Speech and language skills
- Gross motor skills
- Fine motor skills

For each of these, we will first examine descriptions of the types of problems that can occur. Then we will discuss which professionals do remedial work in each area, and when it is important to refer. Last, we will look at things that you can do to help the student with these issues.

SPEECH AND LANGUAGE

Because dyslexia is by its very nature a language-based issue, why is it then necessary to have a separate discussion of this area? The answer is that some students with dyslexia can have severe and distinct problems that require additional intervention. These can be in the following areas:

ARTICULATION

As children are learning to speak, it is normal for them to mispronounce sounds and to substitute some sounds for others. If they do not respond to proper modeling and gentle correction, however, articulation may be a particular problem area. There can also be issues with the quality of the voice, as regards the pitch and tone.

Some students have difficulty pronouncing multisyllabic words. They can say two or three syllables correctly, but then either mispronounce or reverse the remaining syllables.

Stuttering is the perseverative repetition of sounds. This is not a common correlate to dyslexia.

EXPRESSIVE LANGUAGE

Some students can pronounce individual words correctly, but they can't always recall a particular word, and they stumble when they need to express themselves in sentences. They know what they want to say, but their language is not fluent. Sometimes, the speech will be slow and labored. This condition is often called expressive aphasia.

To be truly fluent with conversational speech, a person also needs to be able to use correct grammar. He must have absorbed and be able to use clichés and other verbal conventions. One indication of a serious expressive language disorder is a student's inability to engage naturally in conversation. Notice if he is unable to "give and take" verbally, even when he is in nonacademic settings with his peers.

RECEPTIVE LANGUAGE

Receptive language affects the student's ability to understand and absorb information. A student with a weakness in this area, a condition often called receptive aphasia, can find it difficult to listen. He can be confused by normal conversation as well as by oral instruction.

He can also have trouble understanding directions, especially those with multiple steps. In other words, a direction like "Please close your book and place it in your desk" has two steps. When the student does not respond to the second part, "Place it in your desk," he can be perceived as resistive.

CAUSES

What causes these difficulties? Articulation problems can be caused by a physical problem such as a distortion of the mouth, by difficulty with auditory discrimination (the ability to hear the small differences between sounds), or by poor habits. Issues with expressive and receptive language can be the result of poor auditory discrimination and/or auditory memory, or of a general weakness in phonemic awareness. It is generally believed that neurologically based organic issues are the cause of both receptive and expressive aphasia, although more research is needed.

Most students with speech and language issues have normal hearing. Of course, there are exceptions, and all students should receive hearing screenings. It is also important to find out if, as a young child, a student had a lot of ear infections. This can create intermittent hearing loss, which can interfere with his acquisition of language because he has lost valuable "hearing" time. Even older students who are prone to ear infections can still experience temporary hearing loss due to this physical condition. This is very important to check out, because medical intervention may be necessary and, if appropriately provided, can assist the development of language.

Speech and Language Therapists

Speech and language clinicians provide direct services to students with significant issues. If you are concerned about a student, ask to speak with a speech therapist. Sometimes, a preliminary screening form can help determine if more formal evaluation is necessary. Speech and language clinicians can work directly with students. They can also provide support in both special education and regular classrooms.

Hints

Use the following suggestions for helping students with speech and language issues:

- Check to see if there is a language other than English or a distinct dialect spoken at home or in the student's community. Inform the speech therapist about this.
- Be aware of how many steps your student can understand and follow with oral directions. Be careful that you limit your steps to this number.
- When oral directions and instruction are being given, try to create as distraction-free an environment as is possible.
- See if there is a place in the room where your student seems more attentive to oral communication. Speak with him about this and let him sit in that spot when oral instruction is being presented.
- After oral directions have been given, check in with your student to see if he has understood what was said. Make a plan for him to use a simple gesture that can alert you that he is confused.
- Speak in complete sentences as much as is possible. In other words, say "Would you like to do some reading now?" instead of "Want to do some reading?" Even though the latter is more true to conversational speech, it helps the student to hear as much grammatically correct English as he can.
- Notice words that your student mispronounces regularly and try to use these words in your speech. Don't point out his articulation errors, but rather provide a model for proper pronunciation.
- Don't allow your student to be rushed when he is speaking. Other students can sometimes become impatient and interrupt and finish the statement. Speak with your students about this, and insist that all students be given safe and quiet time to finish what they are saying.
- Question your student about the content of what he has said. For example, if he has just said, "My dog had five puppies," you can ask, "Are the puppies active, or are they sleeping all the time?" Often, students who have expressive language problems become used to people not really listening to them. By your question, not only do you tell him that you have heard what he has to say, but you also give him an opportunity for more practice with speaking.

- Find out how comfortable your student is with speaking aloud to other people. Does he never feel good about it, or does he feel okay when he talks with one or two friends? Can he participate in a small group discussion? Try to provide opportunities for him to communicate in a social setting that feels safe, and then expect him to speak.
- Read aloud. Read in a nonhurried and expressive manner, then ask questions about what you have read. As with all situations, however, first make sure that your student feels comfortable in the social situation in which he is being asked to practice speaking.

GROSS-MOTOR AND FINE-MOTOR SKILLS

GROSS-MOTOR

On a school trip where a group of students with dyslexia were climbing a steep rock face, one of the boys was spread eagle on the rock. He became frightened and called for help from his peers.

"I can't move," he called. "I'm stuck."

There's a handhold to your right," his friends called. "Go to your right."

"Where's my right?"

This is a true story that illustrates the far reaching implications of difficulties with gross motor skills. Unfortunately, it is not uncommon for students with dyslexia to experience them.

Gross-motor refers to the large muscle groups in our bodies. When people have difficulties in this area, they are said to have trouble with sensory integration. This is believed to be a neurological condition that is organically based. People are either overstimulated by movement of the muscles in their bodies or understimulated by it.

Some students with dyslexia can have excellent gross-motor skills and can be fine, even gifted athletes. But for the student who has a weakness in this area, organized sports can be a time of fear and embarrassment. Even everyday activities can be affected, like riding a bicycle and playing catch with friends. Poor sensory integration can cause difficulties in the following areas:

Motor coordination. Students can have trouble using their muscles as a team.

Balance. It can be hard to deal with gravitational forces and to keep the body upright.

Directionality. As noted in our story above, the student with this issue really has to think about what is his left or his right.

Sequencing motor tasks. When facing a complex motor task that is made up of several steps, it can be hard to know what to do and how to complete the simpler motor tasks in order.

Knowledge of where the body is in space. This is a lack of awareness of how one's physical being relates to the environment, including both objects and people. It can make the student with this difficulty look clumsy.

Poor muscle tone and strength. This weakness can be further accentuated if the person does not enjoy motor tasks (because he doesn't feel successful) and thus avoids them.

Difficulty crossing the midline. Even though we don't have a specific line down the middle of our bodies, it is helpful to think of both sides working together bilaterally. It is important to be able to cross over the imaginary midline for certain movements.

Tactile defensiveness. This is a hypersensitivity to being touched or a hypersensitivity to touching certain textures. It is a very difficult condition as it relates to social considerations, because it's hard for people who do not experience this condition to understand or sympathize with people who do. Thus, the student is often embarrassed about his heightened sensitivity and is reluctant to disclose it.

A few students with dyslexia have strong dislikes of certain kinds of food. There is much speculation about the cause of this, but it is generally believed not to be an emotionally based eating disorder. It is speculated that the cause may be tactile defensiveness, that the feeling of the food being chewed in the mouth may be creating a strong aversion.

Fine-Motor

Fine-motor refers to the use of the small muscles of the body. This is particularly important as it relates to holding a book and turning pages while reading, doing handwriting, and also using computers and other academic tools. A weakness in fine-motor skills can be a serious impediment to academic success. Specific difficulties can be present in the following areas:

Eye-hand coordination. Students can have difficulty making their hands do what their eyes want them to do, such as copying from the board or from another paper.

Laterality. This is the ability to easily tell left from right, and to use this information automatically while completing motor tasks. Students often have trouble with reverse letters, as with "b" and "d," and "p" and "q," when writing.

The whole issue of laterality for students with dyslexia has been debated a great deal in these past few years. Some people believe that reversals are a common trait, even into adulthood, whereas others claim that this is a myth. They point out that all young children reverse letters and that reversals are no more common among people with dyslexia than any others.

Eye-hand coordination speed. Some students can get their small muscles to do what they want, but they are very slow. For them, handwriting large amounts of text can be extremely laborious.

Planning space. It is important to know where to place text or drawings, both in relationship to the page itself and, also, to the other written elements (words, sentences, drawings). Difficulty with planning space can cause particular problems with written mathematical computation.

Memory for motor movements. Once a person with good motor memory performs a given motor task a few times, the movement becomes relatively automatic. This does not happen for the person with a weakness in this area.This can be a major problem, especially in the area of handwriting, where the formation of letters must be fairly automatic.This is why good handwriting programs for the student with this issue utilize the large muscles to inform the small ones and, also, use repetitive language cues to stimulate motor memory.

Difficulty crossing the midline. As with gross-motor skills, it's important to be able to go back and forth across the imaginary line that runs down the center of our bodies.A student who experiences difficulty crossing the midline will do things like pass a crayon back and forth from his left hand to his right as he is coloring on different sides of a paper.

WHEN TO REFER

Occupational therapists provide direct service and classroom support for students with both gross-motor and fine-motor issues. The title of the specialist is unusual, because we normally don't think in terms of occupations for these skills.An occupational therapist, however, *is* usually the person who is called upon to provide services in the school setting.

You should refer your student for an occupational therapy evaluation if you notice significant difficulties in any of the above named areas. If you are concerned but can't cite any specific problems, it can often help to start a simple log, just jotting down small characteristics that trouble you. Sometimes, there are subtle indications that you half notice in your busy teaching day, and if you keep such a log, a pattern can emerge.

Occupational therapists provide careful and structured remediation as well as classroom support.They notice and work with such issues as how a student reaches and grasps. Does he have tactile awareness, in other words, can he discriminate between the feel of different textures? Can he manipulate an object in his hand, such as clay or a coin? Can he use his two hands together? Can he use such tools as scissors and pencils? The services of an occupational therapist can be very important for some students.

HINTS

Try the following suggestions for students with gross-motor issues:

- Find out all that you can about a student's particular motor weaknesses so that you can avoid activities and games that draw attention to these weaknesses.

- Find out about the sports and games with which your student feels comfortable so that, when it's appropriate, you can provide opportunities for him to move and have fun.
- For the student who experiences tactile defensiveness, try to avoid touching him lightly, especially if this touch will come as a surprise. If you need to touch your student, on the arm with his permission, apply steady and firm pressure. This seems to be an easier touch to accept.

These suggestions are helpful for the student with fine-motor difficulties.

- Keep a chart of capital letters prominently displayed somewhere in the classroom, or give the student a sheet of these that he can keep in his notebook. Even when students are competent with lowercase letters, they can forget what the uppercase letters look like.
- Be aware that fine-motor skills are necessary for computer use as well as with pencils. If an occupational therapist is available, get advice on how to help your student with these skills. It can also be helpful to get advice about proper posture at the keyboard. This can prevent physical problems such as wrist and hand injuries later on.
- Limit the amount of direct copying that is required, especially copying from the board.
- Do not ask students to copy their own work so that they can make it neater. Students with fine-motor issues often make as many space planning and other errors the second time around, and the copying will be a frustrating experience for everyone.
- Have students skip lines on written work.
- Use wide-lined, as opposed to college-lined, paper.
- Provide physical structures for written work. For example, place a small *x at* the beginning of a line where a student is supposed to write. For math computation problems, provide graph paper.
- Limit the length of written assignments so that your student will be successful. Because it requires a great deal of effort for him to write at all, it is more beneficial for him to have a positive and successful experience with a shorter assignment, rather than an exhausting and frustrating experience with a longer one.
- Provide alternatives occasionally. Allow students to do projects rather than asking for written products.
- Sometimes allow oral tests for part or all of an evaluation procedure. This is particularly important for essay portions of tests.
- Allow a high school student, who sometimes has to take notes, to either tape a lecture portion of a class, or team him up with a classroom buddy who will share his notes.

INTERVIEW WITH MIKE

Here, Mike, who is a paramedic and runs his own construction company, talks about some of his experiences with issues with speech and language.

When you were in elementary school, did anyone ever talk with you about your speech?

I had a million hearing tests. They always thought it was my hearing. I used to have a hearing test every week, I think. The person who did it, we became personal friends, because all she does is screening tests.

Do you remember any experiences you had with speaking when you were in school?

Mrs. Bodin made me memorize the Gettysburg Address. I had a hard time with it. You were supposed to do it by Christmas. If you took that class, you had to memorize it. It took me till the first of the year, but I did it. It was hard for me. It wasn't the memorization part; it was pronouncing the words. She used to stop me, and I'd have to start all over again. You had to be precise. You couldn't just mumble the words.

That was one of my biggest challenges at school. It was a great speech, but I didn't see why we had to memorize it. I couldn't get the logic of how it was going to benefit me anywhere in the rest of my life, why I spent so much time and energy when I couldn't even do other stuff. It was frustrating for me. I'm a common sense kind of guy, and she couldn't tell me that.

CHAPTER 14

ADD AND ADHD

Many students with dyslexia also experience symptoms of Attention Deficit Disorder (ADD) or Attention Deficit Hyperactivity Disorder (ADHD). ADD is the difficulty attending to external stimuli in a sustained manner. ADHD has the added component of hyperactivity, or body restlessness.

It's not that the person cannot focus. Think, for example, about the student with ADD or ADHD who sits for hours playing a computer game. She is focusing with great intensity and duration. In fact, it truly seems that she's in her own little world. Her ADD, however, does make it difficult for her to pay consistent attention to something outside herself, for example, a teacher demonstrating a math problem on the board.

Motivation seems to be a highly influential factor. Also, extraneous stimuli such as people passing in the hall, or the heat going on and off, can distract her from the instruction.

Both ADD and ADHD are believed to be neurological conditions. Much more research is needed regarding the cause.

CHARACTERISTICS

The form that ADD will take varies for each individual. The most common characteristics are

- *difficulty paying attention to something that is not innately interesting*, such as verbal instruction or an assigned chore
- *the ability to focus intently for an extended period of time on something that is interesting*
- *difficulty screening out extraneous stimuli* such as background noises and, thus, the tendency to be distracted by them
- *impulsive behavior*, such as acting or speaking before thinking
- *difficulty listening to and following directions*, especially complex ones

- *disorganization with time*, with particular difficulty organizing a work or study schedule
- *disorganization with space*, especially with keeping belongings in an organized way
- *a tendency to lose possessions*
- *inconsistencies in performance, so that functioning is erratic from day to day*
- *poor self esteem*, especially around school work

In addition, students with ADHD can experience the following:

- *Physical restlessness and hyperactivity.* Often, these students are as frequently under the table as they are sitting at it. Their legs move. Their hands are fidgeting, and they talk a lot. Just sitting still requires serious effort.
- *Social immaturity.* They can have difficulty knowing how to act in social situations. Waiting their turn in games, activities, and conversations is a challenge.
- *Issues with self-control*, such as aggressive outbursts and other inappropriate behavior, especially when overtired.
- *Difficulties with transitions*, such as moving from one class to another.
- *Lack of confidence in social situations*, and corresponding frustration with them.

HOW CAN TEACHERS HELP?

It can be overwhelming to consider the list of possible characteristics associated with ADD and ADHD. Each person, however, is unique and usually experiences only some of these characteristics. Also, the degree of severity can vary. Students *can* be helped to cope and to compensate for these issues.

In the next chapter, "Behavior and Social Issues," you will find specific suggestions made for helping the student with behavior issues. In this section, we consider what students with both ADD and ADHD need.

Care and compassion. This is a key factor. It's not that you are a friend to your student, because it's crucial that you maintain the clear boundaries of being her teacher. She does need to know, however, that you care about her as a person, and that you understand that her difficulties are neurologically based. She is not being bad; instead, she is being challenged by a difficult set of symptoms. She needs to know that you are on her side and that you will do anything you can to help her overcome any problems.

Clear expectations for behavior and academic work. The student with ADD and/or ADHD does not tend to guess well. Be explicit about what you require of her.

Consistency. Behavior and academic expectations need to be a firm and safe base from which she can operate. She already has enough difficulty following all the rules. Having the rules change will completely confuse and upset her.

Structure. It is critically important to provide a positive and nurturing structure. Tell your student at the beginning of the lesson what types of activities will occur. Then, follow that plan. For example, for writing, you could say to your student, "This morning, first, we'll write a list, and then we'll work on our paragraphs. Then, at about 10:15, we'll play that noun game you like so much. At 10:30, I'll read to you for ten minutes." Often, it is helpful to develop a consistent structure that will be followed during most lessons in an academic area. This helps the student feel safe, because she experientially knows what will be expected of her.

Interactive and interesting curriculum. Because motivation is a key factor, make real efforts to actively engage your student in her own learning. She learns best by discovering patterns and facts, as opposed to just being told about them.

Variety in the lesson. In a given class hour, for example, plan a lesson that will entail sitting, standing, moving, discussing, writing, and manipulating materials. As one teacher expresses it, "My class just moves faster than they do." It's important to keep each of these activities short and to move naturally from one to another. If you find that your student can focus for a long time on a particular type of activity, plan lessons utilizing that activity for future work.

Student involvement. Your student needs to have a part in planning and creating her own success; she will then be much more motivated and engaged in the activity that is developed. As much as is possible, let her have input regarding subject matter for reports and projects as well as the types of activities for classroom work and homework.

A plan for disengaging from an interesting task. Because your student has a tendency to stay highly focused on something that interests her, create a plan that will help her leave that activity when she needs to do so. Talk about this in advance with your student, and create some signal, either a word or phrase or a physical gesture that will become a familiar and well-recognized sign that she needs to move on. It is often helpful to give an initial verbal cue, such as, "Karen (student's name). Please look at me. Good. We have five minutes left for this activity."

A plan for transitions. Here again, it is helpful to discuss in advance what will happen during a particular transition. Ask your student to participate in the creation of this plan, and keep it simple.

Assistance with organizing space. Take some time to help her set up her work area. Where will she keep her pencils? Books? Then, make sure that there is a physical system in place for helping her keep track of her academic work, such as ongoing lessons and homework. A three-ring loose-leaf notebook, with tabs separating types of papers, can be particularly helpful.

Assistance with organizing time. Make sure that she has a plan for how she is going to approach both work in class and homework, especially long-term assignments.

An awareness of the environment. Your student generally needs a quiet and neat environment. She needs to be relatively close to you so that you can occasionally communicate privately at eye level. If there is a significant environmental change on any given day—for example, if the school yard outside your window is being resurfaced, with heavy equipment coming and going—it is probably most productive to plan a less demanding lesson for that day and to expect a higher incidence of distracted behavior.

Teacher resiliency. It is a common trait for your student to do well one day and to experience frustration the next. If you see failure coming, modify your expectations so that she can be successful. Keep trying different things. If your first plan doesn't work, go on to another and another and then another. Your student needs to know that you are never going to give up on her. You both will just keep trying things until something works (most of the time).

Flexibility. This seems contrary to the high degree of structure and consistency that your student needs most of the time. "Most of the time" is the key phrase, and 95 percent of the lessons should be consistent. Once in a while, however, a day occurs when your student truly seems incapable of functioning. Rather than having a failure experience for that day, quickly change your lesson plan. If you are working with her in a small group or individually, say, for example, "You know, we haven't measured the schoolyard yet for our math project. It's a nice day. Let's do it." If your student is part of large group, try to create an appropriate diversion for her for at least a part of that day. The next day, when your student comes to class, begin as you always have, returning to the consistent pattern.

A relaxed and confident teacher. It is challenging to teach students with attention issues. Seek out support for yourself so that you can have confidence in your approach. Find out as much as you can about your student's specific issues and about what she needs. This information can be obtained from the school psychologist, special education teacher, or administration. If an outside counselor or consultant is part of the team, ask for release-of-information forms to be signed so that you can discuss programming and approaches with that professional. Once you have the information you need, seek out an appropriate support system for yourself so that you can discuss conflicts and issues. Always protect the student's privacy and have these discussions only with people who are on the team and who are authorized to be sharing information about this student. But remember, you need support, even if it is to express frustration and disappointment over not feeling successful on a given day. And you need to share successes. When you say, "Hannah listened for five minutes to my demonstration, and then she started on her project and worked independently for fifteen minutes!" the person who is hearing this report should understand how important and dramatic this progress really is.

MEDICATIONS

Medications are sometimes prescribed for students with ADD and ADHD. These medications should never be the only form of treatment. They are, in fact, most effective when combined with the classroom approaches and techniques listed above. Sometimes, counseling is also recommended.

Two main families of drugs are used. The most commonly prescribed are stimulants, which have been studied and used for approximately 50 years. Some stimulants:

- Brand name: *Ritalin*® (methylphenidate). This drug is usually given two to three times a day, although there is a long-acting form that is taken once a day. The drug starts taking effect within 30 to 90 minutes. It helps people to focus attention and to control hyperactive and impulsive behaviors.

- Brand name: *Dexedrine®* (dextroamphetamine). This drug is similar to Ritalin ® in that it is taken two to three times a day, and takes effect within 30 to 90 minutes. It also helps with attention, impulsivity, and hyperactivity.
- Brand name: *Cylert®* (pemoline). This drug can be prescribed if Ritalin® and Dexedrine® are not effective. It's taken once a day and usually takes a few weeks to affect any improvement in focus, impulsivity, or hyperactivity. A person's liver functioning must be carefully monitored while taking this drug.

A second family of medications used is antidepressants. These drugs can be prescribed if stimulants cannot be used or are ineffective, or in addition to a stimulant if the person is experiencing clinical depression. Antidepressants can help decrease hyperactivity and aggressive behaviors, as well as depression. Common antidepressants that are used:

- Brand name: *Norpramin®* (desipramine)
- Brand name: *Tofranil®* (imipramine)
- Brand name: *Elavil* (amytriptyline)

Most antidepressants take two or more weeks to take effect.

There are side effects to most drugs, especially when first prescribed. For stimulants, these can include headache, irritability, and loss of appetite. Two examples of side effects from antidepressants are dry mouth and confusion. If you become aware of any of these, or of other unusual symptoms, it's important to report them to the school nurse or other designated professional. That person should contact the parents or guardians, who will then discuss the side effects with the prescribing doctor. Sometimes, medications must be changed, or the dosage must be altered.

Sometimes, drugs need to be administered at school. This is usually done by the school nurse or another designated school professional. In this case, it's important to help your student remember when she needs to go take her medication. Because of the great importance of maintaining a regular schedule of drug administration, you should never rely on your student's memory alone. You can have an unobtrusive environmental signal such as, "Go down to the office when the bell rings for the first graders to go to lunch," or you can remind her, if necessary, by a hand signal.

ALTERNATIVES TO MEDICATION

Some parents and students are reluctant to take medication because of the side effects and because of discomfort with drugs, in general. There *are* alternatives that can be considered. Unfortunately, there is not enough research evidence to support the claims of all of them. Also, an approach or technique that helps one student may not help another. The frequently discussed alternatives are examined in this section.

MUSIC

Teachers report that playing certain music in the classroom seems to help with calming and focusing attention and also with transitions. Often, classical music or environmental tapes are played.

DECREASING THE AMOUNT OF SUGAR IN THE DIET

There is a good amount of anecdotal evidence to support the claim that having a student eat less sugar helps decrease hyperactivity. There are other factors involved, however, such as how much protein is also being consumed and when. More research is needed for optimal effectiveness of this approach.

THE FEINGOLD DIET

This diet eliminates food coloring, additives and preservatives. It is strict and difficult to enforce, especially for children. This diet has been proposed as a treatment for ADD and ADHD since 1975. However, many individuals do not propose using the Feingold diet because of lack of conclusive evidence on its effectiveness.

CHIROPRACTIC

Proponents of this treatment approach say that misalignments of the skull and also the spine can cause the body to function less than optimally. Correcting these misalignments will, therefore, help attention and behavior.

SENSORY INTEGRATION THERAPY

This therapy has been developed by Dr. Jean Ayers, an occupational therapist. Because many students with ADD and ADHD have gross-motor issues and some have tactile defensiveness (a repulsion to being touched, which is so severe in some cases that it is uncomfortable to wear certain kinds of clothing), Dr. Ayers recommends specific exercises to help balance sensory input.

BIOFEEDBACK

Neurofeedback is a type of biofeedback in which people are taught how to control certain brain waves so that they can improve their concentration. Current research is suggesting that this form of training may hold real promise, and many people feel strongly about its possibilities. Others question its effectiveness.

RESOURCES

There is a wealth of resources about ADD and ADHD. An excellent catalogue that offers many books and other resources on the topic is:

A.D.D. WAREHOUSE
300 Northwest 70th Avenue, Suite 102
Plantation, Florida 33317
1-800-233-9273
Fax: 1-954-792-8545

Another company that has many books on the subject is:

HAWTHORNE EDUCATIONAL SERVICES, INC.
800 Gray Oak Drive
Columbia, MO 65201
1-800-542-1673
Fax: 1-800-442-9509

Six books that are particularly recommended are the following:

Beyond Ritalin, Facts About Medication and Other Strategies for Helping Children, Adolescents, and Adults with Attention Deficit Disorders by Stephen W. Garber, PH.D., Marianne Daniels Garber, PH.D., and Robyn Freedman Spizman (Harper Perennial, copyright 1996 by Marianne Garber, Ph.D., Stephen W. Garber, Ph.D., and Robyn Freedman Spizman).

The LD Child and the ADHD Child: Ways Parents and Professionals Can Help by Suzanne H. Stevens (John F. Blair, Publisher, Winston-Salem, NC, 1996).

How to Reach and Teach ADD/ADHD Children: Practical Techniques, Strategies, and Interventions for Helping Children with Attention Problems and Hyperactivity by Sandra F. Rief (The Center for Applied Research in Education, 1993).

The ADD/ADHD Checklist: An Easy Reference for Parents and Teachers by Sandra Rief, M.A. (Prentice Hall, 1998).

Power Parenting for Children with ADD/ADHD: A Practical Parent's Guide for Managing Difficult Behaviors by Grad L. Flick, Oh.D., foreword by Harvey C. Parker, Ph.D. (The Center for Applied Research in Education, 1996).

ADD/ADHD Behavior-Change Resource Kit: Ready-to-Use Strategies and activities for Helping Children with Attention Deficit Disorder by Grad L. Flick, Ph.D. (The Center for Applied Research in Education, 1998).

INTERVIEW WITH JEREMIAH

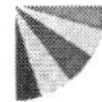

Here, Jeremiah, the 15-year-old student who is so talented in art and mathematics, talks about how he feels about ADD.

When did you first hear the words dyslexia and ADD?

I heard them somewhere around first grade since my dad is dyslexic. I heard my mom talking about how he's dyslexic. I knew that I wasn't very good at reading. It was hard for me and I had to struggle, and I didn't like reading that much, and I didn't know why. But it was probably around fourth grade when my mom told me that I was dyslexic and that's why I didn't like reading and why it was hard for me.

And, then, you know ADD, probably two or three years ago, and Mom explained that, and now it makes more sense why every waking minute, I'm thinking about something, actually more like three things.

Every waking minute, you're thinking about three different things?

Yeah, I never get bored, I just get like, I just have to do something. I'm never bored to the point where I can't think of anything. I can always think of things. It's just that I need to think of things, and I also need to be able to draw or do something with my hands or fiddle with something. I'm always, like, fidgeting, that's the word I'd use, I'm always fidgeting, which is probably why I focused on drawing because it's the kind of thing you can do on the sides of your notes in class. So when it gets really boring, that's what I do.

So what do you think. Do you feel that you have a little dyslexia or more than a little?

I think I have a little of everything. I'd say I'm like kind of between mild and moderate dyslexic. I think I have a pretty big problem. I jump lines a lot. I skip lines and I have to find and go back where I am. I have to use my finger and move it down and move it across the line. That helps a lot. I used to use paper. My spelling is pretty horrible.

Computers are really helpful for school, because I sit down and start typing and spell check comes up and highlights the word, which is very nice. But if I have to write in class, if teachers have a problem, I sit down and explain how I'm a little bit dyslexic, and they usually say, "Oh, no problem." And, in fact, they like to know because they understand me more and they realize why I have the problems.

The ADD is quite mild. I don't have the H in it. I'm not ADHD, which is nice because otherwise I'd run around everywhere. I'm kind of, I just always have to do something. If I close my eyes, I see something. I've never had a night when I haven't dreamed. It's kind of like, I can never turn off, which is nice, because it makes me think of things. I like to think of ADD and dyslexia and dysgraphia and motor output problems as benefits because since I have all those things, the right side of the brain is stronger . . . like I'm good at drawing.

What's hard for you about having ADD?

In school, it's like lectures and sitting down. I was talking before about how I have some disabilities in one side of the brain, but the other side of the brain is gifted? Well, that other side for me includes art and math. I get in math class, and things kind of dawn, I don't have to even think about them. They'll pop, boom, they're out there, and I can just keep going on and on.

If I'm in a math class that isn't challenging enough, it's like—my math class now is enjoyable. It's challenging, with a lot of new information, and I enjoy it, but every now and then, there will be something that my sister will have told me about, or it will be review, or the class isn't getting it.

When we slow down, I kind of get to the point where, it's like they slow down, so I fall off a cliff because I'm running along the edge of a cliff because I'm moving and the cliff slows down, and I'm still moving faster, and so I hit the point and whoops, it's too far, and I kind of flump and I don't know what to do and I draw or doodle, but that's not what I want to be doing. If it's a math class, I want to be doing math. I can't convince myself that this isn't a math class, that this is drawing time. I want to, like, get up and talk to the teacher.

What's nice is that the last few years, I've had a really smart kid in my math class. He's really nice, and what he does is he challenges me.

Math is one area where I can get a lot out of it. If I don't get my release from life, I crash.

The release is the stimulation?

The release is the stimulation of being challenged. With my ADD, my brain always has to be doing something, and if it's like two percent of my brain listening to a lecture, I don't like it. If I'm using my whole brain for something, I love it. I get so enthralled in it. My brain is like being starved the rest of the day for information. I get to the point where there's a banquet laid out for me (with math), and when the banquet is gone, I'm still hungry. And so, it's really nice to be at the point where I don't have to be making stuff up for my brain. Something else is feeding my brain.

So most of the time, you're stimulating your brain.

Yeah, I'm either thinking of a story that I'm making up, or I'm thinking about math problems that I'm going to do. It's nice to have somebody else give you the stimulation.

Do your friends know about your ADD?

My best friend knows about all my ADD stuff, and he thinks that, he says, "For you, it's perfect. For me, it wouldn't be because if I had dyslexia, I wouldn't be able to do social studies as well as I do, which I love doing," He says that he feels glad for me. He doesn't feel envious, because he doesn't want it, but he thinks it's the best thing that can happen to me—that means that I can draw very well, which he can't, and I can do math very well.

He sees that I can go on and on and argue with professors about math and that he can't. He's one of the people who has trouble with the class, so he loves it, so he thinks it's a real advantage.

CHAPTER 15

BEHAVIOR AND SOCIAL SKILLS

COMMON CAUSES AND MANIFESTATIONS

Some students with dyslexia have positive and productive social and academic behaviors. Others, however, do not. One or a combination of the following can cause issues with behavior:

- Organic and/or neurological factors that make it difficult for the student to control impulsive, aggressive, and hyperactive behavior
- Emotional factors, such as feelings of failure, shame, and discouragement, which make it hard to sustain effort
- A lack of knowledge of the appropriate ways to act
- A tendency to misread social cues such as body language

The most common behaviors that can negatively influence a student's academic and personal growth are

- Impulsive and aggressive acting-out behavior
- Withdrawn, isolating, and passive resistive behavior
- Off-target behaviors, such as a lack of responsiveness or a seeming insensitivity to social cues

We will first introduce three fictional students, each of whom exhibits behavior primarily from one of the above categories. Then, we will list some ways that teachers can help.

A STUDENT WITH IMPULSIVE AND ACTING-OUT BEHAVIOR

Let's call him Miguel. He's eight years old, in second grade, and his dad is a carpenter. Miguel loves to help his father. His dad reports that Miguel is a great worker. He'll carry materials to the building site and hammer nails and do whatever needs to be done. "He'll work from morning to night," his dad reports, "and he learns by watching me. I don't have to tell him too much."

At school, Miguel gets along well with his teachers and peers when he's in a small group. In the large classroom, however, he's as much away from his desk or under it as he is sitting properly at it. He blurts out answers and interrupts people during instruction. He tends to tease his peers, poking them or playing with their things. At recess, his teacher is likely to hear "Miguel took the ball. He won't play the game right." "Miguel hit me." When Miguel is asked to come inside early from the playground, he is angry and upset.

"He's such a sweet little boy when he's with me alone," his teacher says. "I don't know why he can't learn to get along with his peers."

A Student with Withdrawn, Isolating, and Passive Resistive Behavior

Paula is in sixth grade. She lives with her mother and father and two younger sisters. Her parents own a landscaping business. Paula's father reports that he has to walk with her to school every day, to make sure that she actually enters the building.

Paula is a quiet student who tries to choose a seat in the back of the class. If her teacher is not watching her or interacting with her, she often puts her head on her desk and takes a short nap. Paula consistently seems tired and withdrawn, except at recess. During that time, she and two or three of her buddies grab a ball and enjoy a rousing game of soccer. At recess, Paula looks like a healthy, happy kid.

A Student with Off-Target Behavior

Tony is in eighth grade and lives with his mother in a third-floor apartment. He's a computer whiz and can spend hours playing games. Recently, he's discovered an interest in creating software. Tony says that he doesn't need friends, because most kids his age are boring.

When Tony was observed during an art class, he was sitting at a large table with four other students, making free-form pottery. When someone asked him to pass the water jar, he did so without comment and made no eye contact. When asked what he was making, he stated, "A jar."

"It's pretty," a girl said.

"It's a stupid project," Tony said. "I don't know why we have to do them."

Tony seemed not to notice the looks that passed between his fellow students. When he finished his jar, he got up from the table without speaking. He left his extra clay for the others to clean up.

HOW CAN TEACHERS HELP?

What do all these students need in order to develop more positive and productive academic and social behaviors? In the following section, we will list some of the things that you can do to help. We will begin with the factors that are always important and then discuss some interventions which are beneficial to some students.

THINGS THAT STUDENTS ALWAYS NEED

Appropriate Instruction. This is listed first, because this is the cornerstone of positive behavior management for the student with dyslexia. Once a student feels safe and successful in his academic program, his nonproductive behaviors often decrease in intensity and frequency.

Positive reinforcement of appropriate behaviors. This is the second cornerstone: Praise. Praise. Praise. Praise *good efforts* and *real accomplishments.* Praise briefly but frequently, and praise behavior that you can observe. For example, it is more effective to say, "Karen, it's terrific the way you shared your pencils with Mary." It is less effective to say, "You're great. You're a great kid." The explicit praise clearly informs the student about what she is doing right and will often motivate her to repeat it.

At times, you have to be very observant in seeking a behavior that you can truly praise. It is important, however, to find a positive one, even if it is only brief and intermittent, because the praise has to be genuine—and immediate.

Reinforcement of positive, not negative, behaviors. "But I never reinforce inappropriate behavior," a teacher says. "I tell him over and over to stop that fidgeting and to sit still." It is important to limit and to have firm consequences for negative behaviors, but your main emphasis should not be on them. In the prior case, for example, the teacher is, in fact, reinforcing the fidgeting, because she is focusing upon it. The student is getting a great deal of attention from his high activity level. It would be far more effective for the teacher to ignore some of the fidgeting and, when he is resting quietly (if only for a moment) to say, "Harry, look at how well you're listening. Good for you."

Establish clear expectations. It's best to have only a few rules and to keep them clear and simple. Make sure that your students understand all of them. In many cases, it's best if students can participate in the development of these rules. For some students, it helps to record these rules, either in a notebook or on a large paper in the classroom.

Provide consistency. Consistency creates safety. The lack of it creates confusion and impulsive and other negative behaviors.

Provide a well-organized and structured classroom environment. This should relate to both physical space and time.

Provide predictable outcomes, including fair consequences for negative behaviors. It's helpful to have a warning system, such as an agreed-upon gesture or spoken phrase, which will alert the student to his negative behavior. If he continues, you should inform him of the consequence in a firm, calm voice.

Provide a sense of caring. Most students profit from the feeling that their teacher cares about them, but this is especially true when negative behavior is being addressed. Provide many opportunities for private conversations about how things are going. Students with dyslexia really need this personal approach. This is not a frill, or something to be done "when there is time." This is an essential element of helping a student develop positive behavior patterns.

When you talk with a student, give him plenty of time to say what he wishes. If he is reluctant to express himself, accept this, but still offer him opportunities in the future. And you can say how you feel; you can tell him what you are observing, especially noting the positive behavior and academic progress that he is making.

If you are concerned about something, you can express this from a personal viewpoint. For example, if you notice that your fifth-grade student is always sitting at the edge of the playground during recess, you can say, "I notice that you spend a lot of your time alone during recess. I think that you may not feel comfortable playing with the other kids." Just express your opinion, and give your student time to discuss it further if he wishes.

THINGS THAT STUDENTS SOMETIMES NEED

A home-school connection. Students (and parents) sometimes need frequent, ongoing communication with the school. This can be accomplished by a weekly phone call, or by a daily note that the student takes home. If you write a note, it is critically important to report only positive behaviors. If the student is having a really difficult time, ask for a meeting of the team or discuss the problems in a parent-teacher conference. The notes should report only accomplishments and successes.

Direct teaching of social skills. Knowing what is acceptable and what is not can be extremely important. As seen in the story of Tony, a student with dyslexia can sometimes have difficulty "reading" social cues. Tony is an extreme example. Many students with dyslexia, however, have some problems in this area.

They can have trouble recognizing what body language, such as facial expressions, means. Often, they don't communicate what they intend to with their own body cues. They can also have trouble recognizing and respecting other people's personal spaces and boundaries. Establishing eye contact when relating to others can be an issue.

How can you help? First, contact your school psychologist or school counselor for some guidance. Make sure that the professional is part of the student's team and that you can freely exchange information about the student's program.

With this support, notice the social behaviors with which your student has particular difficulties. Choose one to work on. This can be either the most accessible one that can be easily improved so that your student will feel successful, or it can be the behavior that is the most destructive and needs intervention the most.

First, talk with your student about the specific social behavior you wish to teach. Obtain his input as to how he feels about this. Then, model the appropriate behavior. For example, if he is always invading another person's physical space, you can demonstrate the appropriate distance that you would keep your body from another person. While doing this, talk about how people like to feel that they have a sense of privacy and control around their own bodies.

Some things that often need to be focused upon are

- reading body language
- expressing feelings and opinions with body language
- reading people's physical boundaries
- establishing eye contact

- beginning a conversation
- maintaining a conversation
- active listening
- dealing with disappointment and frustration in social situations

Opportunities to practice productive behaviors. As with most learning, students with dyslexia can profit from the practice and review of positive behaviors.

A direct intervention plan. First, gather the team to discuss the behaviors that are impeding your student's social or academic progress. This team can include the guidance counselor, school psychologist, school social worker, school administrator, other teachers such as the art teacher, the student, and the student's parents or guardians.

With this team, prioritize the behaviors. If a student has multiple issues, it can be overwhelming for him and for you to try to mediate all of them at one time. Therefore, it's important for the team to choose one or two behaviors upon which to focus. Create a plan, which will be consistently carried out by all present, on how you will deal with these behaviors.

The following helpful techniques can be considered in the development of your plan.

A contract system. With your student, clearly outline the behavior with which you are going to work. Be specific about what you are observing now and what the new, more positive behavior will look like. For example, if the target behavior is sitting at a desk and beginning an independent paper-and-pencil task, you could say something like the following. "Right now, I notice that when you have an assignment, you often get up and get a drink of water. Then, I observe that you wander around the room for a few minutes. What we're working for is for you to be able to sit right down and get your pencil in your hand and start writing. Are you willing to work on this?" If the answer is yes, ask your student to write what the positive behavior will be on a piece of paper. For example, "When I get seat work, I will sit right down and begin working."

Next, discuss positive consequences for successful new behavior. It's recommended that these positive reinforcements be nontangible, such as

- free time
- computer time
- time with a special game or activity
- the chance to work with some special art materials
- being able to substitute an assignment of the student's choice for a teacher-directed assignment

Write out what you will do once the student has been successful with the new behavior for a specified number of times. For the example listed above, you could write, "Once (student) has sat right down and gotten to work on his independent work on 5 occasions, I will allow him to have 30 minutes of free-choice time." If the contract system is to be effective, the reinforcer has to be something that the student really desires. Once the statements are written, you and the student should sign and date the contract.

The following is a summary of the elements of a successful contract approach:

- Be specific about the old behavior.
- Be specific about the new behavior.
- Be objective and nonpunitive while discussing both.
- Ask your student to write down what the new desired behavior will be.
- Write down what the positive reinforcement will be.
- Student and teacher both sign and date the contract.
- Keep checking that the reinforcement is desirable to the student, and change it if it is not.

Time-out periods. Some students become overstimulated by the noise and activity in the classroom, or by their own internal stimulation. This is especially true if the student is tired. Time-out should be a preventive, nonpunitive approach.

In advance, discuss with your student his occasional need for some quiet time alone. Create a plan with him in which *he* can ask for this, or *you* can signal him to go to the time-out area for a specified amount of time. Five to fifteen minutes is usually a good amount, depending upon the student's age and needs. Make sure that the time-out area is truly private and quiet, so that it will provide the lowered level of stimulation that your student occasionally may require.

A cueing system for avoiding negative behaviors. Often, a student can be unaware that he is exhibiting a negative behavior. For example, he can be concentrating on his reading while his legs are knocking the table leg repeatedly. This type of behavior can be annoying to peers, and thus it is especially important to help him become aware of it.

Speak privately with your student about one or two behaviors that he wishes to learn to control. Examples of these can be excessive talking, interrupting others, fidgeting with materials, moving legs or arms, or grabbing objects. Together, decide upon a signal that you will give when you notice him not controlling himself. This can be either a gesture, such as a hand signal, or a word or short phrase.

Take special care to discuss how the student will become aware of your signal; you want this to be a relatively private occurrence, of which his peers are unaware. If you are going to give him a hand signal, for example, you might agree to first say his name and make sure that he is looking at you. Verbal cues should be given privately and at close physical proximity. In this case, you might touch the back of his hand to gain his attention. Preventive cueing can be especially effective if all adults who interact with the student use the same cueing system.

Behavior modeling. Some students need to be shown what appropriate behavior looks like. If your student has difficulty with paying attention to verbal instructions, for example, try to seat him next to two or three students who attend well. If he tends to interrupt others in conversation, sit with a small group of students and tell them that you all are going to practice listening well to each other. Tell them that you will be discussing a specified topic, and that the most important thing is that all the students have plenty of time to finish what they wish to say. Watching others practice this skill and practicing it with them can be very powerful.

Provide a safe plan for handling strong emotions. Students with dyslexia can sometimes be overcome with feelings of anger, frustration, or disappointment. A major goal of your program is to avoid this, but occasionally a social situation or unpredictable academic expectation can arise. An example of the latter is a special guest or teacher who comes into the classroom and unknowingly places an expectation on your student that is unattainable. In spite of your careful efforts to avoid situations such as this, they can happen in a busy school environment.

What your student needs most is a plan, discussed well in advance. What will he do if he finds himself terribly embarrassed, and he wants to run out of the classroom? What will he do if one of his peers tells him that he's not reading "real" books, and he suddenly feels like punching him? Will he approach you quietly and, with an agreed upon signal, tell you that he needs to go to a time-out area? Or will he ask to be able to walk once or twice around the school building? Or does he need to go to the school nurse's office, where he can rest for fifteen minutes?

If you know that your student occasionally has difficulty handling strong emotions, discuss the various options for dealing with them in advance. *He* may create the best plan for himself.

A NOTE ON PASSIVE RESISTIVE BEHAVIOR

Teachers tend to focus on aggressive and impulsive behaviors, because these are very obvious. The student who is passive resistive is usually quiet, and he tends not to affect the classroom environment as much as the active, attention-seeking student.

The passive behavior pattern, however, can mask a great deal of anger, fear, and disappointment. It's difficult to maintain a stance of "I don't care, and I wouldn't do this work even if I could." Most students want to succeed and to cooperate. To pretend not to requires a great deal of effort.

As with the more overtly acting out student, be honest with your student about what you see. Then, try to provide as safe and successful a learning environment as is possible. Once your student sees that he can be successful with academics, he is likely to be willing to make the effort.

WHAT STUDENTS DO NOT NEED

We've discussed many of the elements that help students learn and practice productive behaviors. The following list tells you the things that you should not do. Each one of these can seriously harm a student's progress.

- Don't change the rules.
- Don't "give in" on a consequence "just this one time." Consistency in discipline is essential.
- Don't argue or discuss. If a student tries to engage in an argument, simply and calmly say, "*If* you finish your assignment, *then* you may work on the computer." Repeat the "if-then" statement, until your student really understands that this is the way the classroom is functioning.
- Don't give your students a lot of "don'ts" (for example, "Don't get a drink of water during class. Don't sharpen your pencil until you really need to. Don't talk so much). The student needs to hear many "do's." Focus on what the student needs to do, not the negative.
- Don't remind a student of something negative that happened the day before. Even statements like "I'm glad to see that you look happier this morning than you did yesterday" are destructive. Every day is a new beginning. Every day is yet another chance for your student to be brilliantly successful.
- Don't get angry; get support. It can be very tiring to work with behavior issues. Make sure that you are getting what you need in terms of professional support from the other members of the educational team, so that you can—every day—be consistent, calm, and cheerful.
- Don't expect yourself to be perfect. Everyone makes mistakes, and you might raise your voice, or not notice a signal from a student who is requesting your help. If something like this happens, acknowledge it to your student and apologize. This will build your relationship. He knows that he's not perfect. Now he knows that you aren't either, and this will help him feel safe and comfortable with you.

INTERVIEW WITH THOMAS

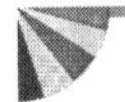

Thomas is attending classes at a literacy program for adults, where he is now learning to read and write. He speaks more about his experiences in Chapter 20.

What was it like getting along with others when you were a kid?

I used to get in a lot of fights. They used to pick on me, because they used to call me dummy and stupid and laugh at me. When I got in about the fifth grade, things started changing, because they stopped laughing and everything, because they found out that I wasn't the only one. There were a lot of others who couldn't get the schoolwork, like about one third of them. It wound up being quite a few of us. They could help a couple of us, but they couldn't get all of us caught up.

Did you have friends?

I always had friends. I had friends that I grew up with, but they were in the same boat as me. They couldn't read or write that good, either.

I never went to any school dances or things like that. 'Cause though they accepted me, I still felt like an odd ball. And sports, it wasn't my thing. I could tell them anything about a car—but sports, it wasn't my hobby.

CHAPTER 16

SELF-ESTEEM AND OTHER EMOTIONAL NEEDS

One of the major factors that can make dyslexia so hazardous to the development of positive self-esteem is the hidden nature of it. A student—let's call her Anna—seems so bright, so alert, so curious. She knows so many things. This is not a person who has limited potential.

Anna stared mutely at books in the early grades, trying to please for the first couple of years, but then becoming sullen and withdrawn. She must be lazy, her teachers thought, or perhaps there was an emotional problem. She was, after all, sometimes disrespectful, and prone to sudden fits ot anger.

All that Anna knew was that she couldn't learn to read and write like her peers. Reading all those letters and numbers seemed easy for her friends. To her, they were confusing masses of changing shapes. Every time she looked at them, she felt as if her mind was going blank.

AN ANALYSIS OF THE PROBLEM

EFFECTS ON ACADEMIC LIFE

The most obvious reason for the difficulty with development of positive self-esteem for the person with dyslexia is the high amount of failure that she experiences in academic settings. Many young children with dyslexia are happy and confident before they enter school. Some of them *do* have developmental immaturities, as in the speech and language, physical, or social dimensions. They may be active children who need a lot of structure. By and large, however, most of them also show great promise and good potential, and expectations for their success in school are high. Like Anna, they are alert and curious. They want to relate to the world and to others; they are, in fact, "normal."

Then they go to school. Most of the time, they are immediately confronted with an educational methodology designed for the dominant learning style, which is completely different from their own. They try. They fail. They try again. After many such failures, they decide that they are stupid and they give up.

Even the students who are lucky enough to get early appropriate intervention, probably had to deal with failure initially. By the nature of many schools, all children are instructed in the same way in the beginning. Only those who fail are referred for evaluation and possible intervention.

Several other factors make dyslexia particularly harmful to the development of positive self-esteem. One of these is the aforementioned high expectations. Students with dyslexia seem bright. Why can't they learn like their peers? They must not be trying, lazy. There must be something terribly wrong with them.

People with dyslexia are usually so aware and observant; they are painfully cognizant of how their academic performance compares with that of their peers. Their friends can learn their twenty spelling words each week. They can read and understand the assignment on the board, and they even raise their hands enthusiastically to take their turn to read aloud. The student with dyslexia often spends her school day looking for ways around problems. If she cowers low enough at her desk, perhaps her teacher will forget to call on her to read. And those spelling tests!

One student with dyslexia reports that he used to spend hours at home memorizing strings of letters. So if the spelling words were, for example, "cat," "table," and "cup," he memorized, "c," "a," "t," "t," "a," "b," "l," "e," "c," "u," "p." For some reason, he was able to memorize the letters in that way, but he was not able to remember the spellings of individual words. His system worked fine, until one day when his teacher changed the order of the words as she dictated them for the test.

This example leads us to another important factor that makes dyslexia so hard to bear: People don't understand. How could someone be able to memorize long strings of letters, but not be able to memorize the spellings of individual words? It's true that he could remember the string only for the week of the spelling test, and then it would be gone . . . but still it doesn't make any sense. Teachers don't understand. Parents and peers don't understand. Worst of all, the student with dyslexia doesn't understand. She decides that there *must* be something deeply wrong with her.

Another factor that makes dyslexia hard to bear is the erratic nature of it. It is not clearly understood yet why this happens, but some days the student can perform at a much higher level than she can on other days. It is speculated that there are neurological causes, and emotional factors may also be involved. But the truth is: A student will be understanding and remembering a concept one day, and will be incapable of this the next. Not only is this highly disappointing to her, but also teachers can become frustrated and angry if they don't understand what is happening. Teachers can decide that the student is lazy and "not trying, because she got it yesterday. What's wrong with her today?"

Another aspect of the erratic nature of dyslexia is that more advanced concepts can be easier for the student to learn than less advanced ones. In other words, things that are relatively easy for other people to learn can be devastatingly hard for the person with dyslexia. She can understand advanced philosophical arguments, but she can't remember her phone number. Even dialing numbers on the phone is hard. She can memorize details of complicated designs and paintings, but she has limited visual memory for the spellings of words.

These surprising strengths can lead to high expectations. The surprising weaknesses can lead to low ones. Both, if not carefully examined and discussed, can be damaging.

Effects on Social Life

Dyslexia can also have an impact on a person's relationships. This can be caused by several factors. First, people with this condition are sometimes developmentally immature. It is common for this immaturity to be approximately two years. Thus, if your student is eight years old and in third grade, she can be more like a six-year-old socially. Therefore, her social functioning and interests are more like a first grader's. This can make it difficult for her to make and keep friends in her classroom.

A second factor is the tendency for some people to misread social cues. This inability, discussed in Chapter 15, makes it hard to recognize physical boundaries and, also, much of the social information that is passed via body language. What *does* that facial expression communicate, for example? Is the other person angry or only surprised? If a person has a tendency to misunderstand what another is expressing, then it is almost impossible to communicate effectively.

Other common correlates to dyslexia can also create impediments to social functioning. Keeping track of appointments, being on time, keeping track of a borrowed possession—all of these can be problematic. The person with dyslexia can also have difficulty remembering multistepped directions. This can make her appear either lazy, disinterested, or incompetent when, for example, friends are just asking her "to do two or three things as a favor." Giving or receiving directions to a particular destination? Both can be impossible.

Another major factor that can hinder social interaction is lack of verbal fluency. Some people with dyslexia speak beautifully, expressing themselves flawlessly and easily. Others, however, have word-retrieval or other issues, and their speech is at times halting and strained. They can speak very slowly, or at times use the wrong word. Their use of proper grammar can be faulty, and they can misuse clichés. They can develop habits such as hand wringing while speaking.

Unfortunately, people often judge one another by the fluency of their verbal communication. The language problems, therefore, can be a real hindrance to the natural and easy development of relationships.

All of the factors listed here can make developing and maintaining relationships difficult. They therefore can have a direct and profound impact on how a person feels about herself.

HOW TO HELP

Positive Feedback

The most important thing to do is to focus on the hopeful and positive. It was necessary to outline the major areas of difficulty in the previous section because we first need to understand the issues in order to address them. Sometimes, however, when these difficulties are laid out, they seem overwhelming and insurmountable. They are not. People with dyslexia are usually resilient, creative people who have many strengths. There are many ways around a problem, and you can help your student with dyslexia to find them.

The following are some specific ways to help:

First, and most important, provide appropriate instruction. The most effective way to help a student develop positive self-esteem is to provide experiences in which she can achieve real success. Even if the successes are tiny steps, they are a different emotional experience; they tell the student that she *can* learn, that she *can* complete the tasks she's asked to do, that she *can* have a reason to celebrate.

Provide direct instruction for reading social cues. This is discussed in some detail in Chapter 15.

Listen. Create opportunities in which your student can talk freely and openly about feelings and concerns.

Make sure that in every class period your student can utilize one or more of her strengths. As teachers, we're often so concerned about what a student can't do, that we focus all of the instructional time on this area. It is important to address weaknesses, but our students also need to experience being good at something. Perhaps she is even at a higher functional level in this one area than her classmates who have more traditional learning styles. Just a little time spent in an area of strength will provide great encouragement and energy for all the hard work with the weaknesses, not to mention encouraging the development of positive self-esteem.

Tell your student what she's doing right. Praise her efforts as well as her accomplishments.

Help her set realistic goals, and celebrate the attainment of each one of them. An example of a goal for one week could be, "I'll have my pencil sharpened and be sitting at my desk ready to work at the beginning of math class every day this week."

Seek out an area in which your student is successful outside of school, and express interest in this. Give her a chance to tell you about it.

Make sure that your student understands about her learning style. First, ask her what she knows about dyslexia, and listen carefully. Often, her beliefs can be individual and unique, and quite different from what you imagine them to be. Then, talk about the facts. When you provide information, do it simply and in small amounts. Plan on several sessions to discuss the many concepts presented below. Your student is living life as a person with dyslexia. Many of these factual statements can have poignant emotional significance for her. She therefore needs time to absorb the information.

As with academics, always review what you've talked about before. Ask your student what her understanding is about a particular issue. Then, go on to present a new concept.

Stressing Key Points Regarding Dyslexia

These are key points that she needs to know:

- Dyslexia is believed to be a learning style that people are born with. They do nothing to cause it.
- If a person has dyslexia, there is nothing wrong with her brain. The only difference between her brain and some other people's is that she needs to learn some things, like reading and spelling, with a different method.
- Many famous people, like Winston Churchill and Albert Einstein, are believed to have had dyslexia.
- Dyslexia is not contagious. It is now generally believed to be a genetically based condition, which tends to occur in families.
- Dyslexia is not just about reversals. It is believed to be primarily a language issue, which can affect phonemic awareness and processing, and many other areas.
- If a person has dyslexia, she can have different levels of the learning style. She can have just a little or a high degree of dyslexia.
- Dyslexia affects each person differently. Some people with dyslexia have difficulty with reading. Some do not.
- There are some common weaknesses; for example, spelling is generally a challenging task, even though people with dyslexia *can* learn to be competent with it, especially when they learn to use a spell checker on a computer.
- There are often significant strengths associated with dyslexia. These are commonly excellent creative thinking, the ability to see patterns in a mass of data, the ability to concentrate and focus intently on a challenging and interesting task, and artistic and musical talents. Does your student know what some of her strengths are? If she does not, you will help her to discover them.
- People do not grow out of dyslexia. Your student can learn to read and write and spell and do math and all the other academic subjects. She can find ways to either learn other skills, or learn how to cope and compensate for her difficulty with them.
- (For your older student) Learning a foreign language can be hard. It's important to talk with her guidance counselor and other supportive people about her dyslexia when she is faced with such a task. Some colleges waive language requirements for students with dyslexia.
- (For your older student) Timed testing, and formal testing in general can be difficult. When faced with such challenges, she should talk with her guidance counselor and other supportive teachers. Modifications such as time-and-a-half, untimed, or oral tests can often be made.
- (For your older student) She *can* go to college. She may need some support and some special accommodations, but she can be successful with higher education.

In fact, some students with dyslexia, once they reach college, succeed brilliantly, because they can finally choose to work and study in their area of strength and interest.

- Most important for all students of all ages: SHE IS NOT STUPID. SHE EXPERIENCED FAILURE BECAUSE THE WRONG TEACHING METHODS WERE USED.

It is very important for your student to have that information. It is also important for parents and other professionals to understand it. As much as is needed, talk about dyslexia with them.

Sometimes, it can be helpful to talk with your student's peers and to explain to them some of the learning style differences. You need to be very careful about this, however. Your student's right to privacy and confidentiality is foremost. If this type of "group talk" is being considered, it first needs to be carefully discussed with your student and with her parents or guardians. Your student may want her privacy maintained. It may be important to her to tell whom she wishes about her dyslexia, and no one else.

BOOKS ABOUT DYSLEXIA

Another effective way to help is to provide books about dyslexia. For older students and adults, the following are recommended:

- *In the Mind's Eye: Visual Thinkers, Gifted People with Dyslexia and Other Learning Difficulties, Computer Images and the Ironies of Creativity* by Thomas G. West (Prometheus Books, 1997). This nonfiction book profiles several famous people with dyslexia and also discusses in depth the issues and the strengths associated with the learning style.
- *Reversals: A Personal Account of Victory Over Dyslexia* by Eileen Simpson (Houghton Mifflin Company, 1979). This autobiographical account poignantly records Ms. Simpson's struggles and triumphs.

One piece of fiction that is recommended for younger students is the following.

- *My Name is Brian* by Jeanne Betancourt (Scholastic, Inc., 1993). This story tells the tale of Brian who, on the first day of school, writes his name incorrectly on the chalkboard. Fortunately, his teacher recognizes this and other classic symptoms and refers Brian for evaluation. In his sixth-grade year, Brian learns a lot about dyslexia and, also, about friendship.

SOME POTENTIALLY HARD TIMES

Two particular trouble spots in the school experience can harm a student's self-esteem. One of these is the evaluation time. "Why am I being tested?" your student asks. "What's wrong with me?" Assure your student that there is nothing wrong with her, and that the testing is being done because you are aware that the teaching methods that have been used are possibly not the best ones for her. She is being tested so that her learning style can be checked out, so that you and her other teachers can plan effective and efficient ways to teach her.

"But none of the other kids are being tested. That mean I'm different," she says.

"You *are* different" you can reply. "Every single person in the world is different and unique. Other students need other things; for example, some people need glasses and others need to sit in the front of the room. We want to find out what you need so that you can become excited about learning."

"But why do I have to be tested *again?*" your student says at her three-year evaluation time.

"You've done so well," you can answer. "We need to make a record of your progress. We also need to check out if you need any modifications in the way we are teaching you. You've grown up a lot in the last three years. You may need something different now than you did three years ago."

When approached in a positive, honest way, evaluation time can be an opportunity for your student to realize that her teachers care about her, and that they are being vigilant in making sure they are teaching her well. Some students want to know the results of the testing. Others do not. If your student asks, assure her that you and the person testing her and whoever else she wishes, will be able to sit down and discuss the results at the conclusion of the evaluation. Keep these explanations simple and clear and, as with all conversations with young people, listen carefully to what she is really asking. She may not want a detailed description of all the scores. She may really want reassurance that she's made good progress.

A second potential trouble spot is the time when all students are being given standardized tests. The requirement for this may have been waived on your student's Individual Educational Plan (IEP). Or she may be allowed to take the test untimed, or with time-and-a-half. Whatever the modification, what this says to your student is that she is different.

As with the evaluation issue, reassure her that she is a unique person who has unique needs. Just because she is not taking the test with the rest of the class does not mean that there is anything wrong with her. There is nothing wrong with her. She is absolutely fine. Her dyslexia affects her in ways that make standardized tests unfair to her. Therefore, the school is making modifications, so that a fair testing of how much she has learned can be made.

A third issue must be discussed—the issue of the label itself. Some parents are reluctant to allow a child to be tested, because they feel that if she is found to have dyslexia, she will be labeled forever. "People will look at her differently," they say. "The label will limit the expectations the teacher will have of her. They'll think that she'll never be able to succeed."

Unfortunately, there is some truth to their fears. Some people do not understand dyslexia, and it *can* affect the way they relate to the student. The answer to this dilemma, however, is to deal directly with the myths and lack of understanding. The answer is not to deny evaluation and appropriate instruction if it is needed. If the student with dyslexia does not receive the help she needs, she will deal daily with failure. She will have little chance of succeeding. This ongoing frustration can be far more damaging to self-esteem than an occasional less-than-positive interaction.

Negative interactions with others are damaging, and they should be confronted. One way to do this is to speak with the person who seems to have a lack of understanding. In a calm and objective way, explain what dyslexia is. Often, the person will change her behavior once she has been given accurate information. If she does not, you need to speak with your school administrator about the problem.

Another way to help is to talk with the student herself about peoples' misunderstandings. First, make sure that she knows all of the relevant facts about her learning style, which are listed in this chapter. Then, talk with her about the myths and misunderstandings. In this way, she will be prepared either to speak with the person who is not relating appropriately or to tell you about the negative encounter so that you can intervene. At the very least, she will not internalize the myths, because she will clearly know that the person who is expressing them has a lack of understanding.

HOW TO TALK WITH STUDENTS

There is an effective way to talk with your student about issues and concerns. Arrange for a private and quiet place to talk. Then, when you both are in this safe place, tell your student clearly what you wish to talk about. Limit your conversation to one major concern at one time.

Ask her first if she has anything that she wishes to say about the subject. If she does not, calmly and clearly tell her what you have observed. Be specific about this and cite observable behavior. In other words, it's more effective to say, "I notice that you always have lunch in the corner by yourself." It's less effective to say, "You don't seem to have any friends." To the latter, your student can simply state, "Yes, I do," and your attempt to help her is over.

When you talk with a student, it is also extremely important to respect her privacy. If she doesn't want to talk about something, you should abandon the topic. You can express your opinion. You can say things like this: "I'm concerned about you, because I notice that you put your head on your desk a lot in the afternoons. I think that you're tired. I think that the work in the afternoon may be too hard."

Ask her what she thinks about what you've just said, or ask another leading question. If your student doesn't continue the conversation, that is the end of it. She will, however, know that you care enough about her to notice her and the problems she is experiencing. She will also feel more free in the future to talk with you. With young children, especially, this can often happen at odd times, such as when walking out to the bus or doing an art project.

WHEN OTHER HELP IS NEEDED

At times, students need to talk with counselors, social workers, school psychologists, other psychologists, or psychiatrists. Your student may need therapeutic intervention beyond what is typical for most students with dyslexia. She may be experiencing high degrees of anxiety, anger, and/or depression because of her feelings about her learning style. In addition to her dyslexia, she may also have other issues, such as difficulties at home.

If you observe behaviors that indicate that your student is continuing to have low self-esteem, or that she has significant mood swings or is sad or angry or anxious quite frequently, ask to talk with an appropriate member of the student's team about these behaviors. If no such professional is involved, tell your school administrator about your concerns.

It often helps to keep a log. Quickly jot down any behavior that is worrisome and record the date and time of the occurrence. Often, after a week or two, a pattern emerges. With these specific incidents recorded, you can be much more confident talking about why you are concerned.

INTERVIEW WITH HELEN

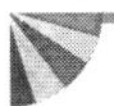

Here, Helen, who was interviewed in Chapter 1, continues to speak about how she feels about having dyslexia.

How do you think dyslexia has affected your life?

Well, I think it gave me a strong feeling that I wasn't very smart for years and years. And I still have to struggle with that. I feel that my children are all smarter than I am. I feel that my husbands have all been smarter than I. Now I make a conscious effort to say, "Okay, there are different kinds of intelligences," and in fact, I never doubt my judgment about things. Sometimes I should, but I don't. I know that I have some good intelligence there, but I don't ever feel that I'm intelligent.

You know, I'm living an ideal life, so I'm not bent out of shape by that sort of thing, but it surfaces.

I think where it bothers me the most now is that I'm aware, more so and more so, that I haven't tried, that I've given up trying. When my grandchildren were learning about dinosaurs, I thought, well I probably could do it if I put my mind to it, could learn the names of the dinosaurs, but I never did. And that made me feel, still does, makes me feel ashamed, because I feel I could have. I could have done that.

How were you made to feel different as a child?

I think more of incidents in later years, when I used the wrong word, and it was funny to other people, but it left emotional scars. Once, I was describing going to Newport, during the Vietnam War. There was a police cordon around, and I said "cauldron," and I remember my friend who was extremely intellectual correcting me, not at all in a put down way. But I felt so unbelievably stupid.

And I avoid words. I mean, just now, I didn't like to tell you that story, because I was afraid I'd make the same mistake over again. And that type of thing haunts me.

The time with the friend, I was beginning to be aware of dyslexia at that point, and beginning to be aware that I had some disadvantages because of it. But, essentially, my judgment is that I'm stupid, and there's no question about that, and what I have to do is hide it. And I will hide it in different ways. I will not talk. I won't try. Now, I really push myself to try things, but for a long while, I wouldn't try things.

If you had the power to choose whether or not you had dyslexia, do you have a sense of what you might choose?

Well, I don't want to live my life over again, but if I could get rid of it now, I would like to. I'd like to live the rest of my life without it, but you know, I don't want to change the past. In the first place, one can't, but if I could learn to spell now, I'd like that.

Do you want to say anything else that you feel is important?

I think maybe that some of the people with dyslexia, especially when it isn't gross—I mean, mine was not gross—have sort of said to themselves, "What I would have to do to overcome this is more effort than I want to make."

I think that's what my son did. He got so that he could read. He still can't spell. And he said, you know, "If I had gone on with it, or if it had been caught earlier, it would have been a lot easier." But in high school, it was very hard to go for tutoring when other people weren't, and he was small for his age so that made it even harder. But I think that it was sort of a conscious choice on his part. He said, "I could get beyond where I am but it would take a humongous effort, and I can get by." And I think that that's a reasonable thing.

On the other hand, he is forever saying to his children, "Practice. It's very important to practice. Everything you do, you have to practice," and I think he feels that he didn't, and he wants his children to learn the value of keeping at something.

CHAPTER 17

TRANSITIONS

Transitions can be times of challenge for anyone, and they can be especially complicated for the student with dyslexia. Both internal and external factors are involved. Concerning the former, the student with dyslexia is often insecure about his academic competencies. Will his new teachers be knowledgeable about his unique learning style? Will the educational methodology employed be effective? Concerning the latter, there *will* be new demands placed on the student. He may be expected to keep track of his possessions and to structure his time more independently. In general, less support may be offered.

In this chapter, we will first discuss the issue of remediation versus accommodation. It is vital that this issue be considered during all transitions, because at these times, a student's program is generally reexamined. Decisions are made about levels and types of services that will be provided. Once we have discussed this important issue, we will look briefly at several critical times of transition.

REMEDIATION OR ACCOMMODATION? OR BOTH?

In remediation, basic skills such as reading and writing are taught. The student's weaknesses are addressed in an individually designed program, which directly addresses his learning style. In accommodation, the student is being taught, generally in a group, with a curriculum designed for traditional learning styles. Modifications are made, such as extra support or variations on expectations.

The first and most significant consideration of which type of intervention is indicated (remediation or accommodation or both) is the student's level of need. Has he, for example, now learned to read and to comprehend well at grade level? But is his reading speed still slow? Can he now form letters, but is he just beginning to write coherent and grammatically correct sentences?

At times of transitions, it is critically important to have accurate and complete information concerning a student's functional level in the basic academic skills. If the student's three-year evaluation does not coincide with the transition time, it may be necessary to do some additional educational testing. Also, talk with his current teachers to see how he is functioning academically and socially in a group setting.

Be optimistic about how well a student will deal with the challenges of a new setting, but be aware of his academic and social needs and plan well for them. Some of the important questions concerning remediation in upper-grade settings are very practical ones:

- When will the remediation be provided if the student has a full class schedule? Will he have to go to tutoring after school?
- Will the tutoring interfere with extracurricular activities such as sports and clubs?
- Will the student be exhausted having to deal with the demands of both regular classes and remediation sessions?
- If he is receiving remediation during the school day instead of a regular class, how will he gain his academic credits?
- Where will he go to receive remediation? Will this be provided in a school setting?
- Who will pay for the remediation?

Accommodation also poses questions:

- Will the accommodations be so obvious that they interfere with the student's social relationships with his peers?
- Should the accommodations be discussed with the class, or should privacy be maintained?
- How much input should the student have regarding the level and type of accommodation made? Some students, especially those with mild degrees of dyslexia, prefer to try to cope with traditional curriculum without accommodations.
- If there is an accommodation such as untimed or time-and-a-half testing, who will administer the test? Where and when will it be administered?

Examples of accommodations that can be made are the following:

- Students can use tape recorders to tape oral lectures or presentations.
- A trusted peer can share notes on lectures and class presentations.
- Taped audio textbooks can be used. More specific information is provided in the following section.
- Homework expectations can be modified with regard to the amount and level of reading and writing required.

- Students can be given different types of homework assignments, such as projects and oral presentations.
- Standards for perfect spelling and grammar in written work can be modified.
- Students can be allowed to use computers for written work in class.
- Tests can be administered orally.
- Tests can be untimed or time-and-a-half.

Many students with dyslexia need both accommodation and remediation throughout their school careers. These two types of interventions should be seen as supportive of and supplementary to each other. They can be most effective if jointly planned by special education and regular education teachers.

The degree and type of this programming will, by necessity, vary as each transition is made. Plan carefully, and assess the effectiveness of the new intervention plan at regular intervals.

RECORDING FOR THE BLIND AND DYSLEXIC (RFB+D)

One accommodation deserves special mention, because it can be a significant help to the student with dyslexia, especially as he makes the transition into the upper grades and college.

RFB+D is an organization devoted to providing audiotapes of textbooks. It was originally started in 1948 to record textbooks for veterans who wanted to go to college but who were blinded in World War II. Approximately three years ago, the organization changed its name from Recording for the Blind to Recording for the Blind and Dyslexic to reflect its expanded mission to include students with learning differences.

The organization recommends that a student with dyslexia listen to a tape as he reads the printed word. It's believed that this process improves comprehension. It also greatly increases the speed of reading, which can transform the reading of textbooks from a slow, agonizing process to a much more efficient and enjoyable one. As part of a well-developed remediation and accommodation plan, recorded textbooks can be a great help to students.

Some recorded books are available at the fourth-grade curriculum level. More books are available for the older grades, with many standard college texts provided. Individuals can also ask that specific texts be recorded. This usually takes some time—approximately three months.

Either individuals or school systems can sign up to receive tapes. There is a fee, although efforts are made to assist individuals who have financial need. For more information about RFD+B, call 1-800-221-4792 or visit the Web site at http://www.rfbd.org.

THE TRANSITION FROM ELEMENTARY TO MIDDLE SCHOOL OR JUNIOR HIGH

The onset of middle school and junior high school varies, but this new placement can be made anytime from fifth through seventh grade. The biggest change is that the student is no longer in a self-contained classroom with one main teacher. Some elementary schools do have team teaching, where one teacher might teach math for all the grades and another might teach reading, but even with this system, the student still "belongs" in a particular classroom.

Most middle schools and almost all junior highs, however, have much more movement from class to class, and individual teachers focus on particular subjects. The student, therefore, has to deal with getting himself and his supplies and homework from place to place. He has to arrive at destinations in a certain amount of time. He has to deal with a wide variety of teachers—along with innumerable distractions—as he moves from one class to the next.

In some school systems, the children are kept in small neighborhood schools for the primary and intermediate years but are then moved to regional and larger schools for the middle grades. A student, therefore, has to learn to manage in an entirely different social situation. No longer is he in classes and recess and lunch with other children whom he has known all his life. Now, there are different kids—unknown kids—and lots of them.

This time of transition also corresponds to the emergence of preadolescence. Some students with dyslexia can be slower in reaching these milestones, so individual students need to be watched carefully as they develop. When a student is solidly in preadolescence, however, this creates some special challenges. A major one is that preadolescents often want more independence. A student with dyslexia who needs a great deal of support from adults can feel resentful about this.

How to Help with This Transition

- Talk with your student. Ask him about his concerns regarding the new placement, and tell him your concerns.
- If possible, visit the new school to see what types of challenges your student will face. If this is not possible, talk with a teacher in the new school about the setting.
- Find out if your student will have any of his friends in his new classes. If not, speak with professionals at the new setting about this.
- Set up a system for daily homework. A homework notebook in which each assignment is recorded can be helpful.
- Make sure that someone "walks through" the new school with the student. Try to arrange a quiet and relatively private time—during the summer perhaps—

when your student can have a tour of the building. If he's expected to use a locker, have someone help him practice with this system. Find the cafeteria and the gym. If possible, let him hear what the fire drill sounds like and go over the procedures for this occurrence.

- Make sure that all professionals in the new setting understand your student's particular learning style. You can ask the school administrator to facilitate the forwarding of relevant information.
- Make sure that there is a contact person to whom your student can go for help if the need arises. This can be a special education teacher or a guidance counselor. A relationship such as this can prevent many problems from developing.

THE TRANSITION TO HIGH SCHOOL

Entering high school is usually the time when adults become concerned about how well a student is doing. Grades count. Achievement counts. Now, it seems more worrisome if a student is well behind his peers in academics. He will, after all, in four short years, be expected either to enter the world of work or to go on to advanced studies. How will he cope if he's still reading at a fifth-grade level?

Remember that students with dyslexia can make significant academic progress during their high school years. Sometimes, their progress begins to accelerate because their physical and intellectual development reaches a level where the remediation can be more effective. Thus, it's crucial to continue significant remediation if the need is indicated.

The onset of adolescence is also a major aspect of a student's high school career. This can be particularly hard for the student with dyslexia, because he wants to do things on his own. He doesn't want to have to ask for help, or to go for tutoring after school. His friends don't need the extra help. They join the track team or the school band or the math club after school. Or they go to a friend's house and "hang out."

Some high schools also have requirements for students to take a foreign language. This can be very problematic for the student with dyslexia, especially if the language is taught in a rapid, nonsystematic way. Issues with weak auditory and visual memories can cause learning a foreign language to be extremely difficult. As one student said, "I have enough trouble with English. I don't want to confuse myself with another language."

How to Help with This Transition

- As you do with younger students, talk with your student. Let him express his concerns. Express your own.
- If possible, visit the high school so that you can see, firsthand, the new challenges and supports.

- Advocate for continued remediation if it is needed. The team meeting is a good place to express your beliefs about what your student needs.
- Ask your student to come to his IEP or other planning meetings. By law, students of 14 years of age or older should be invited to attend.
- Ask your student how much information he wants passed on about his learning style to the teachers at the high school. Some teachers, such as his English teacher, need to know. Does he, however, want only his academic teachers to be informed?
- Ask your student if *he* would like to give information about his learning style to his teachers, instead of automatically having a guidance counselor or special education teacher do so. Would he like to do this jointly, in a special meeting with a teacher?
- Arrange a private tour for your student during a quiet time, such as summer. Explain the most important systems such as fire drills and class schedules.
- Ask that there be a contact person to whom your student can go if he is having difficulties. This can be a guidance counselor or a special education teacher. This can be particularly helpful if your student meets the contact person in advance.
- If the class schedule is a rotating one (if he has different classes on different days), write out each day's schedule for him for the first few days of school.
- If a foreign language is required, try to match your student's particular learning style with the teaching styles of individual teachers. If, for example, your student has a relatively good visual memory and there is a Latin teacher who teaches slowly and methodically while utilizing a great deal of structure, this might be a good match. In some places, sign language is being taught as a foreign language, and that might be an excellent choice for a student with good spatial skills. In some cases, language requirements can be waived on IEP plans.
- Make sure that your student has time in his schedule to pursue interests and strengths. If, for example, he is a talented actor and Drama Club meets every Wednesday after school, perhaps he could miss tutoring for that one day.

THE TRANSITION TO TRADE OR TECHNICAL SCHOOLS, COLLEGE, OR OTHER ADVANCED STUDY

Students with dyslexia often go on to advanced study, either in vocational areas or in academic ones. This is where they often begin to show their strengths, because they are finally able to select the area of interest in which they wish to work. As they make this important transition from high school, however, they need to pay attention to certain pitfalls. Expectations for organizational and academic skills can be high in advanced programs. There will probably be much less support for day-to-day functioning.

For this reason, the law has become involved. Amendments to the Individuals with Disabilities Education Act, first discussed in Chapter 3 of this resource, mandates that students in special education be helped to achieve their life goals through appropriate transition plans and services. According to the 1997 revision, these transition services are to be included on a student's IEP starting at 14 years of age. They can include vocational assessment, specialized instruction, and experiences in the community. These transition plans are to be developed for students who wish to enter trade or technical schools, college, or the world of work.

Two other laws are also important. Section 504 of the Rehabilitation Act of 1973, and the Americans with Disabilities Act of 1990 are two civil rights laws stating that people should not be discriminated against because of any handicap throughout their lifetime. Dyslexia is considered a handicap. These laws, therefore, are very important for the older student, because they ask institutions of higher learning to make modifications in programming. The following are some of the modifications they can be asked to make:

- Allow a student to tape-record all lectures.
- Use texts recorded on tape.
- Give support for organizing and writing reports and papers.
- Give support for the mechanics of written work, such as spelling and grammar.
- Give support for computer word-processing skills.
- Vary testing procedures, such as providing oral tests, or time-and-a-half or untimed examinations.

Students who wish to enter college but who need accommodations on the standardized tests that are often required must contact the testing institution at least six months before the date of the test.

Some colleges, on their own, have waived foreign language requirements for students with dyslexia. Others allow substitute courses to be taken. Some colleges also have programs that are especially designed for the student with dyslexia. These programs can be extremely helpful if staffed by well-trained professionals. More discussion about college, as well as other forms of advanced study, can be found in Chapter 20, "The Adult with Dyslexia."

THE TRANSITION TO THE WORLD OF WORK

Hopefully, by the time the student with dyslexia enters the world of work, he has discovered his strengths and areas of interest. These will lead him to a vocational choice in which he can be successful and function with relative comfort and ease. However, certain areas can be problematic. For example, some people with dyslexia have difficulty organizing space or time. They may often be late for appointments. There may be academic weaknesses, such as spelling, that still pose challenges. Probably the best thing you can do to prepare your older student for work is to discuss these issues with him. Talk about the possible problem areas, and discuss compensatory strategies. Thus, when he faces these challenges, he will be more prepared to figure out his own solution.

The two civil rights laws that protect people with dyslexia in higher education, Section 504 of the Rehabilitation Act of 1973 and the Americans with Disabilities Act of 1990, also protect them in the world of work. Again, because dyslexia is considered a learning difference, it is legally defined as a handicap for the purposes of these laws.

These laws are important because they ask employers to make reasonable accommodations for their workers. "Reasonable accommodation" means that the employer should not suffer undue hardship in creating the modifications. Employers can be asked, however, to do things like the following:

- Restructure jobs.
- Modify work schedules.
- Modify training manuals and/or training procedures.
- Modify testing procedures. For example, if exams are required for certifications or promotions, employers can be asked to provide oral testing, untimed testing, or time-and-a-half testing.

One book that provides more specific information in this area is *Learning Disabilities and the Law* by Peter S. Latham, J.D., and Patricia H. Latham, J.D. (JKL Communications, Washington, D.C., 1993).

INTERVIEW WITH MYA

Mya is a young woman with dyslexia who has just graduated from high school. She will be attending a local community college in the fall.

When did you decide that you wanted to go to college?

Ever since I was young, I always had the idea of going to college.

Why do you want to go to college?

To further my education, and to get a good job. I either want to be a marine biologist, somehow involved in business—like management—or I want to help kids with special needs, mainly learning disabled.

Has your own experience influenced you with this?

Yeah, because I know how hard it is to try to learn, especially when people aren't willing to help you, or to try to find a way. They say, "Well, if you can't learn one way, (Mya shrugs) oh well."

What are some of your strengths?

I'm an understanding person. I take my time with helping people if they need it.

Like my senior year, I was in a special ed study hall. There were other kids who didn't either understand their math or their reading. If I didn't have anything else to do, I'd sit down and help them, no matter what age group: freshman, sophomore, even seniors.

What kind of academic support did you receive in high school?

Well, I had an IEP. I had more time to take tests and more time to finish papers, if I needed it.

Like in my math class, because of the teacher, I didn't understand half the stuff. During that time, if we were taking a test, I'd go to academic support, and somebody would help me the best they could without giving me the answers.

Are you going to ask for academic support at the community college?

Yes. What we're hoping for is to get help editing my papers. Also, I need help with paper structure, because basically I can write my own papers. I just need help to make sure that I'm writing what they want. Sometimes, I'm not sure what they're asking.

We had a meeting at the high school at the end of the year. I believe they wrote a letter to the community college, and to anyplace I go after it. It had my IEP and permission for them to read my records.

Do you know where you want to go after community college?

I'll figure that out later. It depends on what I decide to major in. If I still want to be a marine biologist, I'll go to or near Boston.

What are some of your feelings as you approach entering college?

Nervousness. I'm nervous that I'm not going to get the help that I need. That will make me feel that I'm not succeeding, and that will make me want to give up, or it will discourage me so much, that I won't want to continue. I don't think that will happen, but you never know.

I have a couple of friends who are going to the community college, so that's nice. I have at least one friend that was in the academic support program at the high school.

I'm worried about just getting everything finished in time. And about doing well on tests, because tests with me don't show everything I know, especially if I don't understand the question. That was frustrating in high school, because I could sit down and tell you anything we learned, and then when it came to the test, I'd get a C or D. My friend said, "A C is good. It's average." And I'd say, "It's not good in my eyes."

What are some of your hopes?

I guess getting a job that I'm able to support myself, and that I like.

What was the transition like for you from elementary to junior high school?

I was scared because of my learning disability, but also because I have always been shy, and it's been hard for me to make friends.

How was junior high?

I hated junior high. I had some friends, but I hated the academics of it, and then there was what was happening in my life. My parents were getting a divorce, and it made it hard for me to concentrate on my work.

What was high school like?

I suppose I liked high school. I guess the people . . . I remember when I was in junior high, if they saw a kid going to the special ed room, they'd make fun of the kid. And in high school, there might be somebody who said something, but there'd be others who would quiet him or her.

I wasn't the most popular in high school, because of my shyness, and I have a problem with trust. But if I saw people, I'd at least know them, and they'd smile in the hall and say, "Hi."

What were your teachers like?

There were some who were very understanding, but not everyone. I had one teacher, even when I told her I had dyslexia, she didn't know what that was.

What would you like to tell teachers about dyslexia?

Having dyslexia doesn't mean you're stupid. Teachers should try to accommodate you and find a way to get you what you need. And if you're having difficulties, it doesn't mean that you are lazy. Cause I've had teachers who thought I was lazy. Or if I needed more time on tests, they'd think I wasn't concentrating.

CHAPTER 18

WHAT CAN PARENTS DO?

Parents and guardians play a key role in the emotional, social, and academic development of a student with dyslexia. As teachers, it is important to assist them in that role. We can help parents and guardians in four major ways:

1. Offer suggestions for how they can observe the child.
2. Provide names of resources from which they can learn about the child's learning style.
3. Give specific and practical suggestions for ways they can assist academic growth.
4. Give suggestions for ways they can help in other problem areas, such as homework, and social and emotional issues.

LEARNING HOW TO OBSERVE

A parent is in a unique position to observe a child in a wide variety of settings and times, and to gain and provide valuable information that goes far beyond reporting about a student's early development. When information about what is happening now is shared with teachers, it can greatly assist in the development of an effective educational program.

Many people believe that they naturally know how to observe. There are certain factors, however, that facilitate the gathering and reporting of helpful information.

With the parents, first decide upon the specific area to be focused upon during any given observation period. If you need information in several areas, deal with only one at a time. Choose first either the area that is most troubling or the area that feels easiest for the parents to begin with.

Once you have decided upon an area, write out a series of questions that you would like to have answered. It's often best to brainstorm these questions with parents, having one person be the recorder. Once all the questions are written down, choose one or two that the observer will watch for.

The following are some examples of areas that can be observed, with sample questions for each area:

CONCENTRATION AND FOCUS

- How long can the student concentrate and focus on an activity that is enjoyable and interesting?
- How long can she concentrate and focus on an activity that is not interesting?

ACTIVITIES THAT POSITIVELY ENGAGE THE STUDENT

- Does she enjoy using the computer?
- Does she choose to draw during quiet, unstructured times?
- Does she like to read comics or magazines?

ACTIVITIES THAT CAUSE THE STUDENT TO LOSE FOCUS

- Does she seem not to hear if you speak to her while riding in the car?
- Does she wander off from certain family games?

THE FATIGUE FACTOR

- When during the day does the student get tired?
- When she gets tired, does she need to lay down and rest, or can she just sit quietly by herself for a few minutes to regain her energy?

THE SOCIAL FACTOR

- Does she prefer to be alone, or will she choose to spend her free time with a special friend or with several friends?
- How does she handle conflicts with peers?
- Does she prefer the company of adults to that of peers?

EXPRESSIVE LANGUAGE

- How is her articulation?
- Does she speak using English grammar, clichés and other language conventions properly?
- Does she tend to speak easily, or is she reticent a lot of the time?

Receptive language

- Does she respond quickly to verbal directions, or does she need a physical gesture as a notice to first pay attention to the spoken word?
- How many sequential verbal commands (or steps) can she remember and respond to? (The request, "Please take out the garbage and then put the garbage can in the garage," has two steps.)

Effective Reinforcement

- What types of reinforcement does she respond to?
- Will she work for praise or for free time or for time spent with a special person?

Strengths and Talents

- What does the student choose to do during her free time?
- During what activities does she appear most relaxed and happy?
- In what skills does she seem to be more capable than her peers?
- What is easy for her?

TALKING WITH PARENTS

Once you have established the area of observation and one or two specific questions to be watched for, talk with the parents and decide upon when the parent will set aside some special time for the observation. It helps to be specific about this, because in people's busy lives, time can quickly pass without the observation ever actually occurring.

It's most effective to have these observation periods be short, from five to ten minutes. In this way, it is possible for parents to observe the student several different times and in a variety of settings.

Ask parents to try, as much as is possible, to separate themselves from the behavior they are observing. If, for example, they are watching a child interact with his friend and a conflict arises over the use of a possession, they should not intervene. They should simply watch without the pressure of "having to do something about it." In this way, they will more clearly see the relevant factors in the interaction.

Ask parents to record their observations in a factual manner. In other words, write down what happens, not a judgment about it. For example, it's more helpful to write, "Sally kept playing with her computer game and didn't respond when her sister asked her a question." It's less helpful to write, "Sally ignored her sister." If observing language, it's particularly helpful to record some of the student's actual speech.

After the observations, meet with the parents and discuss the information they have gathered. Take their recorded observations and, together, try to organize them to show clear patterns.

OFFERING RESOURCES TO PARENTS

Parents and guardians need to learn about their child's learning style for many reasons. Probably the most important is for them to be able to understand the child's struggles so that they can interact with her in a positive and supportive way.

Parents and guardians are also the adults who are generally in the child's life throughout her school career. From preschool to transition into the world of work, parents need to relay relevant information. They often are the ones who maintain the vision of what happened before and what is necessary for the child to achieve meaningful and independent adult life. For this reason, they also need information on how to deal with educational institutions.

Resources are mentioned throughout this book. The following are particularly recommended for parents:

To Understand About the Dyslexic Learning Style

- *The LD Child and the ADHD Child: Ways Parents and Professionals Can Help* by Suzanne H. Stevens (John F. Blain, Publisher, Winston-Salem, NC, 1996).

To Communicate with Educational Institutions

- *Finding Help When Your Child Is Struggling in School, From Kindergarten Through Junior High School*, by Lawrence J. Greene (Golden Books, 1998).
- *Negotiating the Special Education Maze, A Guide for Parents and Teachers*, 3d edition, by Winifred Anderson, Stephen Chitwood, and Deidre Hayden (Woodbine House, 1997).
- *The Parents' Public School Handbook: How to Make the Most of Your Child's Education, From Kindergarten Through Middle School*, by Dr. Kenneth Shore (Fireside Books, 1994).

Information on ADD and ADHD

- *The ADD/ADHD Checklist: An Easy Reference for Parents and Teachers* by Sandra Rief, M.A., Prentice Hall, Paramus, NJ, 1998).
- *Power Parenting for Children with ADD/ADHD, A Practical Parent's Guide for Managing Difficult Behaviors* by Grad L. Flick, Ph.D. Foreword by Harvey C. Parker, Ph.D. (The Center for Applied Research in Education, West Nyack, NY, 1994).

About Reading

- *Straight Talk About Reading, How Parents Can Make a Difference During the Early Years* by Susan L. Hall and Louisa C. Moats, ED.D. Foreword by G. Reid Lyon, Ph.D., Chief, Child Development and Behavior Branch, National Institutes of Health, (Contemporary Books, 1999).

About Math

- *Family Math* by Jean Kerr Stenmark, Virginia Thompson, and Ruth Cossey, illustrated by Marilyn Hill (The Lawrence Hall of Science, 1986 by the Regents, University of California).

OFFERING PRACTICAL SUGGESTIONS TO FACILITATE ACADEMIC GROWTH

There *are* things that parents and guardians can do at home that are supportive of good educational programming at school. These activities should never be a burden, however. They should be short, simple, and fun. If there is any strain on either the parent's or the child's part, they should not be continued. The suggestions offered here are obviously not comprehensive; they merely serve as samples of activities that are appropriate to recommend to parents.

To Support Reading Skills

Read aloud to your child. Almost all people enjoy being read to, and listening to a book helps students relate to the written word. A great deal of evidence suggests that reading aloud is extremely effective in helping students progress in their reading skills. This is thoroughly discussed in *The Read-Aloud Handbook: Revised and Updated, Including a Giant Treasury of Great Read-Aloud Books*, 4th ed., by Jim Trelease (Penguin Books, 1995). Reading aloud is beneficial for all ages, so don't stop doing this when your child is older. Find out what type of stories she likes to hear, and read those books.

Create a reading time for the whole family. It's helpful for everyone to just sit together and enjoy their own individual books. Make this a regular time, maybe two or three times a week when everyone can participate. Your child does not have to be reading novels; she can enjoy a wordless picture book or a magazine. Everyone should be "reading" something he or she enjoys.

To help develop phonemic awareness, play rhyming games. Say a one-syllable word, for example, and see if your child can think of a word that rhymes with it. Then, let her challenge you.

To develop the knowledge of letter names, make letters out of cookie dough. Of course, you all have to say what letter you are eating.

Point out print in the environment. For example, if you are driving on a highway and notice an interesting place name sign, just point that out to your child. Read her the labels of tin cans when the labels communicate important information. In a very informal way, show your child how much interesting information the written word can convey.

To Support Writing Skills

Keep a shopping list on the refrigerator. Ask your child to contribute items that your family needs to this list.

Make other types of lists. This is good for the development of word-writing skills. It also supports more advanced writing because it teaches organizational and categorizing skills and encourages the free expression of thoughts into written words. Make lists of a wide variety of topics. Some possibilities are

- things in the living room
- things that are smaller than a nickel
- colors
- things to put in a sandwich
- excuses for being late

These lists can be completed at any skill and age level. They can also be good for long car rides. In that case, even though you may be making the list orally and not writing anything down, you are still practicing categorization skills.

Write a serial story. This is a cooperative story. The first person writes the first sentence to start the story. She then gives the paper to the next person and that person writes the second sentence. This game can be played by any number of players. Students usually enjoy it greatly. They often like to try to change the plot line when it is their turn.

To Support Math Skills

Make math a part of everyday life. The need for math occurs frequently in daily life, and this can be a powerful motivator for students to learn about this subject area. Practical problems can arise everywhere, as in "We've got to buy a gallon of milk and a bag of chips, but we have only four dollars. Will we have enough money?"

Discuss this problem with your child. Complete the mathematical computations yourself, with your child watching. Don't put her on the spot unless she asks to help. As much as possible, create an atmosphere stressing how useful and important mathematics is to daily life.

For children learning number concepts, make associations between tangible objects and numbers. Do this informally, as when you ask your child, "Please give me those two seashells on the table." Make these associations frequently. It's helpful if your child actually touches the objects.

Play all kinds of games, and keep score. Even if your child is not yet capable of doing the computations, model your interest in and enjoyment using numbers.

OTHER PRACTICAL SUGGESTIONS

To Help with Homework

Have a regular time when homework is done. The more consistent this is, the easier it will be to maintain. To establish this regular time, first assess when your child has the energy and focus to work on her homework. Some children do best right after school. Some need to come home and go outside and play until dinner, so after dinner is best. Experiment with a few possible times, telling your child that you are doing this. Then, with her, decide upon the regular homework time.

Establish a regular place for doing homework. Assess where your child works best. Does she need the quiet of her room, or does she function best at the dining room table? If this is the case, should the television in the living room be shut off? Establish a regular homework setting, and stick to it.

Help with structuring assignments. If needed, spend a few minutes at the beginning of homework time looking over your child's homework folder. Help her prioritize her assignments.

Maintain regular contact with the school regarding homework. Is your child bringing all her assignments home? Is all completed work arriving back at school the next day? A simple weekly phone call can answer these questions and prevent other problems from developing.

To Support Positive Social and Emotional Development

Set aside a special time each week when you and your child spend some private time together. You can play a game or go for a walk or go to get an ice cream cone. The time doesn't have to be long. It's most helpful, however, if it's something your child can count on from week to week, because then she will know that she will always have an opportunity to talk with you privately if she so chooses.

If you have other children, make sure that they, also, have this same amount of "special time" each week.

If your child has siblings, talk with her about what she would like her brothers and sisters to know about her learning style. Does she want them to be given lots of information, or does she want them to know only that she learns differently than they do?

With your child with dyslexia present, talk with your other children. Generally, open communication of this type helps everyone feel more comfortable; everyone then understands what is happening both at school and at home.

Talk with your child about what she feels comfortable telling relatives, family friends, and social acquaintances about her learning style. People can ask a wide variety of questions, like the following:

- Why isn't Sarah reading yet?
- Is her speech a little funny?
- Why does she have to go for tutoring after school?
- What does she have? What *is* dyslexia?
- Will she outgrow it?

Talk with your child about possible questions. It's important to elicit from her any questions that she's already been asked or that she is afraid of being asked in the future. Discuss possible answers, and then role play for practice.

Talk with your child about potentially embarrassing situations. Does she, for example, have an uncle who sometimes buys her a book and then asks her to read a page or two? Is this uncomfortable for her? Does your child want you to talk privately with this uncle, or would she like to join you in the conversation? If this is the case, it can sometimes be helpful to role-play a bit, so that your child can practice what she wishes to say.

INTERVIEW WITH NAOMI

Here, Naomi, who is a midwife and is pursuing advanced studies, speaks of her experiences as a mother of a teenage boy who has dyslexia.

Do you think that Malcolm has dyslexia? Is that how you would define Malcolm's learning style?

Well, the problem with using that term is that people think that dyslexia means when you reverse letters, so it depends on who is asking. If it's somebody I'm not going to get into a long conversation with I'll use that term, because it's something that people recognize, even if it's misunderstood. They do understand that it's kids learning in a different way.

Do you feel comfortable with us talking about this in a book that's going to be titled How to Reach and Teach Students with Dyslexia?

Yeah, because my understanding of the definition is that dyslexia really is, that there's a gap between somebody's ability and intelligence and what they're able to do because they have a different learning style.

When did you first discover that Malcolm had a different learning style?

Maybe fourth grade.

And what made you realize it? What happened?

Well, I think it was actually earlier than that because the different testing that they did showed that he had issues with auditory processing. So I would say, early grade school.

What has been the hardest thing for you as a parent?

I think what's hard is that I have a really different learning style from Malcolm's, and so . . . I may be ADD. It wasn't something that was identified. I don't think it was to any extent, so I was able to function, but I need to have things come quickly enough so I don't get bored. 'Cause that's what would happen when I was a kid; if things got too slow, I'd be gone. And that still can be an issue for me. And Malcolm's learning style is more going from one thing to another, more methodically, and I don't have a lot of patience with that.

So Malcolm was lucky because he worked with Martha, and she was so great because she—the way she read and worked with Malcolm—was incredibly methodical and with him every step of the way. But the parent-child thing, it's hard for me to slow down so that I could do that.

So you would like to have helped him more?

Yes. Helping with schoolwork was definitely a hard thing. That's one thing. It's also hard for me to remember that multiple directions are hard for Malcolm to follow, and so sometimes I interpret his behavior as resistance.

You know, if he's getting ready in the morning, and I ask him to do three or four things, it's hard for him to remember all those things. And I go one direction and then come back and he's forgotten some of them. So sometimes he reminds me, but when it comes to pressure around time, or efficiency or patience issues, then it's hard.

Is there anything else that's difficult?

It's frustrating not to know what the possibilities are for the future. So it's fear of the future. And reading is such a interest for me, and where I get a lot of enjoyment. I wish that could happen for Malcolm.

What helps you the most?

I think understanding, that's really helped, and talking with other parents. Malcolm went last spring for six weeks to get some special training, and it was very hard work for Malcolm. Talking with other parents there and hearing the process that they had to go through was helpful. And for me, it's been great seeing that Malcolm has made progress.

And another thing: I took accounting last spring, and I experienced a fog, sort of like being able to get it for a little while and then it would disappear, and feeling how frustrating that was, and how that affected my self-esteem around something that I didn't care that much about. Accounting was really just a requirement. It's not integral to something that I'll have to do. It gave me so much more empathy and compassion for Malcolm. So my own personal experience really helped.

Your own experience of what it must be like as he's sitting there, facing a book.

Yes. That was really helpful. And the same time that was happening was during his special training, and I got to listen to Malcolm working. He works so hard. Malcolm works so hard. I honor his stick-to-itiveness.

CHAPTER 19

TALENTS

It is as important to discuss the area of talents as it is to talk about the weaknesses associated with dyslexia. As teachers, we are often so concerned about academic lags that we focus on those. We sometimes forget to notice and utilize strengths. This is an oversight for several reasons:

- Exercising these strengths is important to a student's academic and intellectual development, because obtaining one skill will facilitate the attainment of others.
- These strengths are important to the self esteem of the student with dyslexia.
- Our society needs these strengths.

A MULTIPLICITY OF STRENGTHS

People with dyslexia usually have significant and strong talents. We can look at the Howard Gardner model of multiple intelligences to gain insight into these. In his book *Frames of Mind: The Theory of Multiple Intelligences* (Basic Books, 1983), Howard Gardner talks about the following different types of intelligences:

- ***Linguistic:*** A facility using language
- ***Logical-mathematical:*** Good ability with patterns and numbers
- ***Spatial:*** Knowledge of spatial relationships
- ***Bodily-kinesthetic:*** Enjoyment and skill with movement and touch
- ***Musical:*** Love of and skill with music
- ***Interpersonal:*** Good social abilities
- ***Intrapersonal:*** Insightful knowledge about the self

People with dyslexia have strengths in many of these areas. There is no clear pattern among individuals; one person is completely different from others. A student with dyslexia can be strong in his spatial intelligence. His bodily-kinesthetic and his musical intelligences can be well developed. These are not compensations for his difficulty with language. Rather, they are reflections of his own unique form of intelligences.

These strengths can often be difficult to see in a school setting, however, because traditional curriculum is based largely on linguistic intelligence. The other intelligences *are* utilized, especially the logical-mathematical one, but there is a bias toward the linguistic; the teacher talks and students listen. Language tasks, such as reading and writing, are presented at rapid speed and with little reinforcement. There is little opportunity for the other intelligences to be explored and to shine.

How, therefore, do we discover our student's strengths? This process of discovery will be our next subject.

THE USE OF INTELLIGENCE TESTS TO DISCOVER STRENGTHS

When intelligence tests were first developed, they focused primarily on the verbal, linguistic skills that a person possessed. Questions were often asked about a person's factual knowledge, and this required him to retrieve and express a verbal label. For example, for the question, "What is celebrated on the Fourth of July?" the person being tested has to be able to remember and state, "Independence Day." He may know all about the holiday, understanding the history and the concepts, but because of a language issue, he may have trouble coming up with the exact words "Independence Day."

As the field of testing has advanced, especially with the advent of the Wechsler tests, there has been a serious effort made to tap skills other than linguistic ones. Thus, Wechsler tests are divided into Verbal and Performance sections, with Performance subtests measuring skills such as attentiveness to visual details, and eye-hand coordination speed. Even with the new generation of tests, however, most are still administered orally, and they are heavily weighted in the linguistic area.

When they are tested, students with dyslexia do not immediately appear to be gifted individuals with significant strengths to offer the world. Their language issues influence their functioning. Their attention, fine-motor, and other issues can also affect their scores.

Yet, a skilled examiner who has a good understanding of the learning style can find valuable information about talents and strengths, especially on individually administered intelligence tests such as the Wechslers. He can notice, for example, on the Block Design subtest in which a person is asked to reproduce two-dimensional geometric designs with three-dimensional blocks, that the student merely glanced at the picture and then created the copy with unusual speed. This indicates good abstract thinking, but perhaps it also indicates skill in the area of sculpture.

Every student with dyslexia is different. Every one has a different constellation of abilities, with a wide range of strengths and weaknesses. This great diversity has created confusion around the nature of the learning style and has made diagnosis problematic at times. It can also make it particularly hard to identify talents, but they are there to be discovered. Intelligence testing by a skilled examiner is a good place to start.

WHAT CAN TEACHERS DO TO HELP STUDENTS DISCOVER THEIR TALENTS?

To discover and name talents, you first need to think about what they may be. There *are* some abilities that are characteristically found among people with dyslexia. The following list includes some of the most common of these.

- At least average, and often, above-average intelligence
- The ability to concentrate intensely and for a long period of time on something that they are interested in
- Great drive and energy for solving problems that trigger their curiosity
- The ability to perceive patterns in a mass of seemingly unrelated data
- The ability to come up with a new concept, a new way of looking at a situation or problem
- The ability to think abstractly
- A high degree of curiosity
- The willingness to ask questions
- The willingness to work hard
- The willingness to take risks
- The willingness to be independent
- A strong sense of humor
- Excellent observational skills
- Excellent spatial skills—the ability to perceive and interact with three-dimensional space
- Excellent mechanical ability
- Excellent artistic ability
- Excellent musical ability
- Excellent athletic ability
- A good sense of direction

Because dyslexia is by its very nature diverse, you will find individual strengths in some students and not in others. Some students, for example, are excellent artists. Others like to fix mechanical things and to create inventions. Still others can be very skilled with computer games, and they can have original and creative ideas for ways to solve problems.

Sometimes, the talents listed above are easy to see. If, for example, a student is talented artistically with drawing and can easily render lifelike pictures, there are many opportunities for this to be demonstrated. In other cases, however, the talents are more hidden. The student who has a talent in certain areas of three dimensional art, for example, and who can create beautiful collages will have fewer chances to demonstrate this skill.

Teachers are in a unique position to name obvious talents and to uncover hidden ones because they interact with the students for a substantial amount of time and in a variety of settings. This is an important first step. Before talents can be nurtured and utilized, they first need to be recognized. The following recommendations can help with this process.

Look for strengths. Focus and observe. This does not have to be a formal and lengthy process. Just notice how your student is interacting when, for example, a visitor comes and asks to use the slide projector. Is your student with dyslexia the person who is the first to offer suggestions on how to remedy the situation when there is too much daylight in the room? Is he the one who is fiddling with and correcting the projector lens focus? Set out to notice strengths, and you will see them. It sometimes helps to keep a "talents log," in which you quickly record any demonstrated abilities. Over time, these quick notes can uncover fascinating patterns of strengths.

Notice areas of interest. Is your student suddenly sitting taller during a discussion of bird migration? Talents are often not far behind interests.

Provide a wide variety of activities. As much as is possible in a busy classroom setting or tutoring time, occasionally offer different types of experiences. Plant some narcissus bulbs, for example, and record the growth of the foliage. Invite your students to create a puppet show that relates to something you are studying. Notice how and with what skill level your student relates to these activities.

Talk with your student about what he likes to do. Sometimes, students have activities that they greatly enjoy at home and never mention at school. As an example, a new student once was presented with a creative writing opportunity. He wrote an original, fascinating vignette full of suspense. His teacher praised his efforts, but then thought to ask, "Have you done this kind of writing before?"

"Yes," he answered. "I write stories at home."

"Have you ever shown them to anyone?"

"No. I keep them in a drawer in my room."

Ask parents about a child's interests and talents. Sometimes, it is important to tell parents that you're not just asking about reading or other academic interests. Some examples of these are

- Fascination and long-term involvement with Lego™ construction
- Hours spent at the computer with a story or adventure game
- A love and concern for animals that is often reflected in wanting to take care of other people's pets during vacations or in trying to find homes for stray animals in the neighborhood

- An interest in gardening, as seen in planting a garden in the back yard
- Hours spent "doodling" or drawing geometric shapes in various perspectives
- An interest in cooking

All of these skills reflect more basic abilities. They also point to future career possibilities.

Ask other teachers about strengths they may have noticed. Has the art teacher, for example, discovered that your student is very interested in watercolor painting? Has the physical education teacher noticed a tendency toward leadership? Has the music teacher discovered that your student plays rhythm instruments very well, especially the cymbals?

HOW TO NURTURE TALENTS IN THE CLASSROOM

First, and most important: Recognize them. Talk with your student and acknowledge his abilities. Ask him questions, and engage in conversation about his areas of interest. One student was a good basketball player and was also very interested in following a particular team. A two minute conversation at the beginning of each day about this sport helped the student relax into the day. It also said to him that his teacher knew him well enough to know what he was interested in, and that his teacher cared enough to ask. Recognizing basketball as a valuable and legitimate interest helped greatly in building a relationship.

Provide opportunities for students to demonstrate their talents in the classroom. If, for example, a student enjoys making birdhouses and has a small business in the summer selling them at the local open-air market, ask him to bring in one or two. Ask him to talk with either a small group or the whole class about how he makes them.

If your student is good at planning and problem solving, ask his opinion about a good system for recycling used paper in the classroom. Perhaps he'd like to create a recycling plan?

If he loves to make aerodynamic paper airplanes and is also a leader, ask him to demonstrate one or two design models in class, and then to organize a contest at recess. The airplane that flies the farthest wins.

The opportunities that you create don't have to be extensive or complicated. They just have to truly tap the student's skills and talents and give a chance for demonstration and practice.

Utilize talents for academic learning like reading, writing and math. In the example of the student who builds and sells birdhouses, see if he would like to read about birds to gain more information. What types of birds are his homes intended for? What are some of the characteristics of these birds? What does the structure of each house tell about the bird's needs?

For writing, would he like to write a list of supplies that he needs to build a particular house? Would he like to write out a series of directions for how to build a house? Or how about a report on his favorite kind of bird?

For math, has he figured out how much it costs him to build each house? How much does each one sell for? What is his profit?

Utilizing talents in this way gets students excited about learning. It also supports and encourages their preexisting interests and abilities.

Utilize talents while remediating weaknesses. This has to be done carefully, so as not to overuse the talent for this purpose. You don't want the talent to become associated in the student's mind with a weakness or "hard work." If used selectively and only occasionally to reinforce learning, it can be fun for students to use their special abilities during remediation. Perhaps, for example, you have a student who loves fabric art. He is particularly interesting in quilt making. If he is working on phonemic awareness, would he enjoy making an alphabet quilt, with each letter having its own square? Your student who loves music might like to create a song for some difficult homonyms he's studying in spelling. Your student who is a fine poet might enjoy writing a poem about a problematic math concept.

Utilizing talents in this way can be fun and motivating. Used sparingly, they'll assist remediation.

Provide opportunities to discover and create new interests and talents. Take that field trip to the aquarium. Invite the grandmother who is a historian and who dresses up as a historical figure and talks about "her life," to come visit the class. Bring in an interesting rock you found in the park last weekend. Have a box full of recycled items in an invention area, where students can create things during free-choice time.

All students, including those with traditional learning styles, profit from stimulation and activities of this type. For the student with dyslexia, however, who has to face work that is difficult for so much of the school day, these activities are particularly important. He needs to become interested in new things, to discover new talents. This will help him keep trying on all that other hard work.

STUDENTS NEED THEIR TALENTS. DOES SOCIETY NEED THEM?

People with dyslexia are among the most creative and talented people in our society. Unfortunately, because of the high degree of emphasis on linguistic skills, especially linguistic skills requiring auditory discrimination and memory, it is sometimes difficult to recognize their great abilities.

When our culture was dependent upon agriculture and hunting, their learning style strengths were very obvious. They were observant, able to find things. They were easily able to answer questions like "Where *are* those fiddlehead ferns that we want for supper?

With the advent of the modern computer age, things are once again changing, and now, some of the skills that are common strengths of the dyslexic learning style are becoming more important. For example, it is becoming increasingly necessary for people in business and other areas to be able to handle large amounts of seemingly unrelated data. The person with dyslexia who has ability to see patterns in such situations will be highly prized.

Many famous people with dyslexia have contributed greatly to our culture. People such as Winston Churchill, Albert Einstein, Thomas Edison and Leonardo da Vinci are profiled in the fascinating book *In the Mind's Eye, Visual Thinkers, Gifted People with Dyslexia and Other Learning Difficulties, Computer Images and the Ironies of Creativity* by Thomas G. West (Prometheus Books, 1997). In this book, you can read fascinating stories about famous people who had great difficulties with linguistic skills. Fortunately, their other talents and skills became apparent, and they were able to contribute a great deal to the world. Your students may enjoy hearing about these famous people, and it's recommended that you consider reading sections of this book during read-aloud times.

What Can Students Do with Their Talents?

Many people with dyslexia become graphic artists, architects, surgeons, and entrepreneurs. Sometimes, it helps students recognize and value their own skills if you point out to them the wide range of career possibilities in which talents can be highly valued. For this purpose, the following list of adult careers is provided on page 318.

People with traditional learning styles also participate in these careers. This list is important, however, to show the student with dyslexia that he has a wide variety of career options. His learning style might make it difficult for him to be an audio tape transcriber, but there are many jobs in which he can succeed. Furthermore, his learning style can help him to be highly successful in these careers.

You might want to share this list with your student, so that he can have fun thinking about future possibilities. Read it with him or to him, and ask if any of the careers sound interesting. You might put a check mark by the appealing ones and then go back and discuss them more thoroughly once you've finished reading the list. Your student might even do research on one or two jobs. The other challenge to offer is to see if he can suggest other interesting careers not mentioned that he'd like to add to the list and explore.

The list is not meant to be comprehensive. It is purposely not tightly organized, but is more of a "brainstorm" list. It is meant to *begin* the conversation about how valuable and important your student's individual talents can be.

CAREER LIST

__ Actor
__ Antique dealer
__ Architect
__ Baker
__ Botanist
__ Cabinet maker/furniture maker
__ Car mechanic
__ Carpenter
__ Cartoonist
__ Cheesemaker
__ Chef
__ Chimney sweep
__ Chiropractor
__ Clown
__ Computer hardware developer
__ Computer programmer
__ Computer software developer
__ Contractor for new homes
__ Contractor for remodeling homes
__ Cosmetologist
__ Costume designer
__ Dairy farmer
__ Dancer
__ Detective
__ Electrician
__ Entrepreneur/restaurant owner
__ Entrepreneur/retail business owner
__ Entrepreneur/service delivery
__ Entrepreneur/wholesale business owner
__ Firefighter
__ Fisherman
__ Forest ranger
__ Graphic Artist
__ Heavy equipment operator
__ Hotel manager
__ Illustrator
__ Inventor
__ Jewelry maker
__ Landscape architect
__ Landscaper
__ Lawyer
__ Logger
__ Machinist
__ Make-up artist
__ Marine biologist
__ Massage therapist
__ Mathematician
__ Musician
__ Nurse
__ Optometrist
__ Painter
__ Painting restorer
__ Paramedic
__ Photographer
__ Physical therapist
__ Physicist
__ Playwright
__ Plumber
__ Political lobbyist
__ Potter
__ Professional athlete
__ Puppeteer
__ Real estate agent
__ Salesperson
__ Sculptor
__ Set designer
__ Social worker
__ Songwriter
__ Store manager
__ Surgeon
__ Tailor
__ Tattoo artist
__ Teacher
__ Vegetable farmer
__ Veterinarian
__ Weaver
__ Welder
__ Wood carver
__ Writer

INTERVIEW WITH RAFAEL

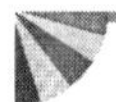

Rafael is a person who has dyslexia. He now runs a cabinet and furniture shop that hires several people. He is very proud that his business has become a supportive community for the people who work there.

Please talk a little bit about what school was like for you as a kid.

School, for me, was a terminal illness that I didn't get over until I got out. School was awful. School, from first to eighth grade, was at the school that my father started and was running, and my mother was the librarian and a cousin was the secretary, and my aunt was the art teacher, and my cousins and two sisters were at the school. So it was a very family filled place.

I had remedial reading help, probably from first grade right up to eighth. The woman was a sweet woman, and I enjoyed going because she fed me jelly beans and chocolate kisses.

Was she helping you?

No. As a kid, I wasn't aware that she wasn't helping me. I was aware that I was having difficulties.

Would you describe your talent—what you think your strengths are?

My strength is manual dexterity and artistic ability. My parents sent me off to summer camp during the summers, and those five summers that I was away helped me get through the winters. And my father had a hobby shop in the basement that I was puttering in and using tools and playing with things.

When people ask me how I became a woodworker, I say four things: God-given ability, we didn't have a TV, my father had a hobby shop, and he gave me my first set of tools when I was seven years old. I have them to this day.

Tell me a little more about your artistic ability.

I'm easily able to see things. I can transfer a set of drawings from two-dimensional to three dimensional in my head. I can take . . . I can look at a set of blueprints and quite easily understand them.

I have a very good friend who is 93 now and who has been an incredible artist all his life. He's so dyslexic that on a postcard, there'll be four or five spelling mistakes. But he's grateful, because he says, "I'm grateful I have dyslexia, because I've got a gift in this other area." He's an incredible sculptor. He's sold 75 percent of his work in his lifetime, and that's unheard of.

When I was growing up, Dad gave me a little workbench in the cellar. In the cellar, each of us five kids had a little work space. And Dad gave me a bottle of glue. Well, that bottle of glue and all the scrap woods under the saw turned into this huge mass of sculpture on my bench that was all glued together. We finally had to take a sledgehammer and knock it all apart and throw it away. (Rafael laughs.)

That sounds wonderful.

Dad insisted that I learn how to use hand tools before he allowed me to use power tools. But I was using power tools—a table saw—by the time I was 10 years old.

What did it mean to you to have this talent when you were a child?

It saved me. I was a failure in school—couldn't read very well, couldn't write very well. I hated school, and to come home to the shop, to Dad's hobby shop, and to spend all weekend down there, all afternoon, whatever—it got me through the terminal disease of school.

What does it mean to you now?

It means that I can support my family. It means that I can support my family doing something that I enjoy doing. I love my job. I love my work. I love the people part, the physical work in it. I now have a shop that has a good reputation. I've been doing this for 26 years.

Was your talent ever recognized in school?

Somewhat, in art class. The teacher was one of my aunts, and she always enjoyed me.

What were junior high and high school like for you as concerns your talents?

I was a leatherworker.

I thought you started woodworking as a child.

Well, I was playing. I was learning and using saws and creating stuff. But the summer before I went off to high school, I saw a guy who came to the camp for the day. He was a leatherworker, and he did a demonstration. And I watched him all day, glued. So I came home and said, "Mom, I want to buy a piece of leather."

And I started making things out of leather, and I very quickly realized that I could make belts and pocketbooks and other things. That part of my high school career was good because I was developing a skill, and a skill that brought me some cash.

After high school, I got out and started working for Tony (a furniture maker) because he knew my talent, or potential. And I looked around and saw that there were so many more things made out of wood than of leather, that I switched my medium and started making things out of wood.

It required very similar skills. They transferred back and forth between leather and wood: measuring and cutting, things like that. Different tools, but it was very similar skills.

When you look back at your life, who or what has been most encouraging regarding your talent?

Probably being given the space to do it. Having a shop, and tools that I could just putter with.

I worked for Tony only for nine months, and then he went out of business for personal reasons, and that left me without a job. So I went to the store that he and I had been building things for, and I said, "Hey, Tony's out of the picture. Can I make these table bases for you?" And the owner looked at me—I was 19 years old—and he said, "Yeah," and he wrote me out a purchase order.

So at 19, you started your own business.

I jokingly tell people that I was 19 and too young to know what I was doing, but I did it anyway. So I rented my dad's shop in the basement for a year, and then after a year, he told me, "Okay, kid, it's time to get out. Go get your own shop and your own tools. Out of the nest." I was still living at home. So we hunted around, and I found a shop, a space that I rented, and I found some tools and I continued my business.

I will say that I couldn't have done it without my wife. The support and love of my wife, who happens to be a special education teacher, has been so important. She understands about my disability. When I started out, I still didn't feel good about myself. I'd walk up to people with my head bowed and give them a limp little handshake.

Now, I stand up straight. I look people in the eye. I have a good, firm handshake, and I'm proud of what I do.

CHAPTER 20

THE ADULT WITH DYSLEXIA

INTERVIEW WITH THOMAS

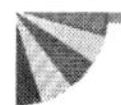

Thomas has been attending classes and receiving tutoring at a literacy project for a little more than a year. He is now learning to read and write.

What was it like for you when you started school?

More or less, they did everything but give me a dunce hat, no matter what I did. I tried to do the work on the board. I didn't care if it was math or reading or writing or science or history. No matter what I told them how it should be, in my words, they told me it was wrong. Because I was behind the desk. The first or second week of school, they put me behind the teacher's desk. It was like I wasn't part of the class. I was in a different class by myself.

Did you have any good teachers?

I had a couple, but they didn't have enough time to go over things with me.

I don't know how anybody could do it, but I flunked first grade. They sent me to second, but after a month or two, they sent me back to first grade. That's when I gave up.

They kept pushing me through, and then when I got to seventh grade, they told me they were going to send me back. But they didn't. Then, I wanted to go to trade school, and the trade school said they would take me. But Ashland (Thomas's home school district) said I had to go back for another year for eighth grade. But I was already sixteen years old, so I said, "The heck with it. You don't want me to go to trade school. You want me to go back for another year. I'll quit." That's when I quit school.

What did you do when you quit school?

I was already working part time in the junkyard. So I stayed working there for the next year or two. Then, they sold the junkyard, and then a guy called me up and said he was reopening a garage near my father's house. I worked for him until I started work for the college, when I was about twenty.

What kind of work did you do at the college?

I worked on the ground crew for awhile, and then I worked as a custodian until I was laid off.

How many years did you work at the college?

Twenty-seven and a half years.

You told me that you've just recently signed up to become a voter.

Yes. Carol (Thomas's teacher) and I filled out the form in pencil. I filled out my address. I had to fill it out slowly, but I got it. I asked a few questions. The words were different than what I'd seen in my own mind.

Are you going to vote?

Yes. They're going to send me more forms.

How did you get your driver's license?

I was about 22 when I got my driver's license. I had a heck of a time. They didn't want to give me an oral test, but they finally did.

How have you gotten by all of these years?

By laughing—that's how I've gotten through most of the time, by laughing. When I first came here (to the literacy program), it was so quiet, it was like a morgue. The first week I was here, I was going crazy, so I started to joke around, cause it's just like me. Whenever I'm around a group of people, I start horsing around. People started laughing and joking back and forth, in a polite way. So Carol said it got to be more a comedy show, but we got to learn things faster and easier. We'd joke about it.

There was this woman, she couldn't count change, so I'd sit with her and say, "Here, count it out. This is better than pencil and paper." And she learned.

What's reading been like for you?

I always read everything backward. I'd look at it, and I'd pronounce it backward. I'd start pronouncing it back to front. I go backward. Nothing ever seemed to click in. It was a blank, a cement wall right in front of me. My eyes were seeing it, but my brain was taking it in the other way or backward.

Did you keep your dyslexia a secret from people in your adult life?

No, I told them. I had people say, "You have to be able to read, the way you seem and do things and talk." But I said, "I listen to everything I come across—news, radio, television."

What are your strengths?

Working on cars. And determination that it's not going to keep me down. Where there's a will, there's a way."

What do you wish teachers had done for you when you were a child?

I wish they had sat down and tried to teach me. But they didn't know any better. They just branded me stupid.

INTERACTING WITH ADULTS WITH DYSLEXIA

In all the other chapters of this book, the interviews have been placed at the end of the chapter. In this chapter, however, the format has been changed to highlight the great importance of the personal history of every adult with dyslexia. We are only now beginning to understand the nature of this learning style, many adults were not given appropriate remediation when they were young. Furthermore, the popular belief when they were children was that seemingly bright students who couldn't learn either were lazy or had emotional problems that were interfering with their functioning.

Dr. Orton and other researchers were already studying the learning style, but their information and theories had not yet been accepted in the wider culture. Thus, teachers of students with dyslexia were given no way to understand the condition or to help their students. They were left to their own individual efforts. Some teachers were more successful in finding helpful ways to teach than were others.

In your role as a teacher, you may interact with adults with dyslexia in two settings. First, if you teach children, your young student may have a parent or other relative who also has the learning style, because dyslexia often occurs in families. This adult's personal history will influence the way she feels about the young person's struggles. It will also influence the way she interacts with the school.

If the adult was treated poorly and with contempt, she may wish to protect the young child, resisting efforts to label her as different. She may want the child to be in nonchallenging classes and to just "get by without a lot of fuss." Another reaction is to deny the existence of the learning style, saying things like "I managed; so should she. There really is no such thing as dyslexia." Or she may be adamant that her child receive appropriate intervention—*now*.

When you interact with these adults, be aware that emotional factors may be highly influential. One way to help is to provide a safe place for the expression of feelings. Also, provide information about the learning style. If you feel that more intervention is needed and that an adult's feelings are negatively influencing a student's chances for appropriate programming, ask for assistance from your school social worker or school psychologist.

The second way that you may relate to adults with dyslexia is to teach them. More and more adults, like Thomas, are seeking this kind of help. Some go to adult basic education programs. Others seek teachers who have knowledge and understanding for tutoring help. Appropriate intervention can be effective at any age, regardless of the degree of the dyslexia. A person who is a beginning reader can be taught, as can the adult who has graduated from college but who is continually frustrated because her reading is slow and labored.

Intervention can be highly successful with adults—partly because they are highly motivated to seek help. Little time has to be spent in motivational or behavioral interventions. Also, any developmental issues that may have been present during their school days will probably be resolved in maturity.

In the following pages, general principles of teaching adults with dyslexia are outlined. The subject areas of reading, spelling, writing, and math are each briefly discussed. The chapter ends with a discussion of college.

GENERAL PRINCIPLES OF TEACHING ADULTS WITH DYSLEXIA

Use the same basic techniques, outlined in the preceding chapters, for each subject area. There is no difference in the underlying principles for appropriate instruction for adults. There are, however, some special considerations and some modifications that are helpful:

When you first begin working, do a thorough diagnosis of your adult student's basic skills. Do not assume that your adult student knows anything. Check. This may seem to be odd advice, because your student may be a highly successful and articulate person. She may have graduated from college or be in a highly demanding field of work. She also, however, may not know the alphabet. She may have been compensating for lack of basic knowledge for years.

Explain to your student what you are doing so that she will not be offended by your assessment. Use a metaphor like the following: Tell her that the basic skills are the foundation of the house of knowledge. If there are holes in this foundation, the house will be wobbly and weak. Filling these holes will make it much more secure.

Provide information about dyslexia. Make sure that your student understands the key points about dyslexia, which are offered in Chapter 16. This knowledge can be critically important.

Provide a little time at the beginning of each tutoring session for your student to discuss anything she wishes. This may be what has happened in her week, or she may have questions about her learning style. Often, this unstructured and relaxed few minutes can greatly help your student enter into the tutoring time in a focused way.

Occasionally, provide conversation openers that invite your student to talk about her school history. Always be aware that she has probably had many negative experiences with academics. She may want to discuss these, or she may wish to maintain her privacy. Follow her lead on this. If she *does* want to talk about aspects of her former education, listen carefully and express understanding and empathy for her feelings. Time spent in this way will help her to move on to successful remediation.

Discuss the theoretical basis for the remediation techniques you are using. Even done briefly, it will help your student understand the focus of her work.

As much as is possible, relate instruction to the person's interests. Adults with dyslexia often have well-developed areas of fascination. Use these. Read books on the topics. Write about them. Use metaphors from an area of interest to discuss educational concepts.

Sometimes, your students will come up with these metaphors on their own. Thomas, who was interviewed at the beginning of this chapter, is fascinated by auto mechanics. When discussing phonemic awareness and how people with dyslexia often need remediation in this area, he related it to his interest and said, "My brain has been in park all these years. It hasn't been in reverse. It hasn't been in drive. Because if it had been in drive, I'd have known all these things."

Ask your student for feedback regarding her remediation plan. Adults are very clear about what is helping them and what is not. At the end of each tutoring session, ask your student if she felt that the lesson was working for her. What, if anything, was most helpful? What, if anything, was least helpful? Does she have any suggestions about other things that might be tried? Adults can offer many valuable insights into optimal programming.

Make sure that your student learns something new during the first tutoring session, and that she learns something specific every tutoring session after that. This may be a fact, such as that there are six or seven (depending on who is counting) types of syllables in the English language. If you are focusing on spelling, you can present the derivation of a common word in every session.

It is a big commitment for an adult to take time out of her busy schedule and to work on something that can bring up a lot of pain from the past. And real remediation—the type that truly helps reading comprehension and writing and other advanced skills—takes time. It helps your student to keep on, therefore, if there is something interesting in every tutoring session that she can bring home with her.

ISSUES INVOLVED IN TEACHING READING

A main difficulty with teaching beginning reading to adults is the scarcity of appropriate reading material. The person who is just beginning to read profits greatly from having a book with pictures, with just a few words of text on each page. It is particularly helpful if the text is of a larger than normal font size. The pictures provide valuable context clues. The limited text seems inviting instead of overwhelming.

Many teachers feel that it is inappropriate to use picture books that are created for children to teach reading to adults. You *can* find some picture books in libraries and book stores that have photographs or other illustrations that are more acceptable because they are less "cute" or childlike. For example, the book *Truck Trouble* by Angela Royston in the Eyewitness Readers Series (DK Publishing, Inc., 1998) presents a story of a truck driver who is making a special delivery. Even though the book was designed for children, it has less of a childlike feel because of the full-color photographs.

If you look hard enough, you can find some of these books. The problem is that beginning readers need to read a lot of them, and there is not a wide variety available. For this reason, some teachers feel that even conventional picture books can be used as supplementary reading material. Talk with your student about it; discuss the issue and see how she feels. Some adults do not even want to consider it; others, however, feel comfortable with picture books, and some really enjoy them.

One very insightful teacher in an adult basic education program made the following comment while watching an adult learner smile and laugh over the antics of Clifford, the big red dog, in *Clifford's Kitten* (story and pictures by Norman Bridwell, Scholastic Inc., 1984). The teacher said, "I guess that, when she was a kid, she never got to sit with a book in her hands and just enjoy reading it. It's nice to see her relax with a book."

One other technique that is very helpful in providing reading material for new readers is to have them dictate information or stories about their lives. These can be written down and then typed in larger than normal font size. Double spacing also helps. This autobiographical material can then be used for the cooperative and cloze reading techniques described in Chapter 6, "Teaching Reading." An example of such a story follows. It was dictated by Thomas, the person interviewed at the beginning of this chapter. It tells about the early life of his daughter.

THE MIRACLE BRAT

She was what the doctors called a blue baby. They never tried what they did with anyone else. When they went in, they found out she had only half a heart, so they had to rebuild it. That's when she was 18 hours old. She was in and out of the hospital for a cough or sneeze or cold for the next $2^1/_2$ years.

The first weekend she was home, four generations were there with her—her mother, her grandmother, her great-grandmother, and her great-great-grandmother; so we took a picture of the five generations.

Then, when she was $2^1/_2$ she went to the Children's Hospital, and they operated again because she was having leakage. At the same time, she was paralyzed on the left side, so she had to stay there longer. She was there 31 days.

The next to the last week in June, she got married, and her grandmother was still there, and her great-grandmother was still there. She is 98. We took a picture of the four generations.

February 15, she will be 21. For a blue baby to be this many years—it's a gift from God.

It is essential to provide structured, multisensory phonics instruction for the early introduction to print, and this work should be continued throughout a student's remediation plan. As people develop their literacy skills, however, it is also very important to encourage them to practice their reading in an area of personal interest. A fascinating article, "Literacy Development in Successful Men and Women with Dyslexia" by Rosalie P. Fink, Lesley College, appears in the *Annals of Dyslexia: An Interdisciplinary Journal of the International Dyslexia Association* (founded in memory of Samuel T. Orton), Volume 48, pp. 311-346, 1998. This article describes a study conducted with 60 men and women with dyslexia. The conclusion of the study is that extensive reading in an area of fascination is a key to the development of high levels of literacy. When people are reading about something they're interested in, they are learning new vocabulary unique to the field, and they are gaining familiarity with the structure of written text. They are reading a lot. They are thinking about what they're reading. All of these factors help develop reading fluency. This fluency can then be utilized when reading text of less interest.

ISSUES INVOLVED IN TEACHING SPELLING

Checking basic skills is critically important. Many adults with dyslexia have particular difficulty with the short vowel sounds. As with younger students, it is important to present these sounds, but it is not necessary to stay only with them until mastery is obtained. Present them long enough so that your student is very aware of them, but then move on to other phonemic elements. Provide consistent practice and review of the vowels.

Computer spell checks can be very helpful for the adult student. Often, however, she needs to raise her spelling level so that the spell check will be effective—so that it will be able to recognize the desired words, and, also, so that it will not select an oppressive number of words. Ability to use a computer spell checker can be an important goal.

If your student has reached the level where she can use spell checks effectively, do some extra work with homonyms. Spell checks don't always discriminate between homonyms, so it is necessary to have some basic knowledge of these words. Sometimes, it's a good idea to have your student do some free-writing at the keyboard. Print out what she has written, after the spell check has been utilized. Then, check the writing for homonyms. In this way, you may be able to pick out some with which she needs extra help.

ISSUES INVOLVED IN TEACHING WRITING

All adults need to be checked out for their word writing and sentence-writing skills, even adults who seem to be able to write longer works such as letters and reports. Practice at these more basic levels can greatly improve writing fluency, the ease with which thoughts are expressed and organized on paper. Writing fluency is a major issue for adults, because many of them have learned to compensate well enough to get thoughts down on paper, but they do so with great struggle and unease. Their writing can be slow and labored, and their basic feeling about writing tasks is often dread.

If work is done at levels below their functional level, however, this negative feeling can begin to change. They can begin to relax around writing.

It is particularly important to spend a good deal of time at the paragraph-writing level, writing structured paragraphs that consist of the following:

- a topic sentence
- three supporting detail sentences
- an ending sentence

Write *many* paragraphs with your adult student, so she will internalize this very necessary English form. Don't stop practicing with paragraphs once she understands the structure. She has to write so many that she relaxes and begins to feel that writing paragraphs is actually quite easy. When she approaches writing a paragraph as just a simple warm-up exercise, then it is time to move on to higher levels.

Once your student is ready to move beyond this stage, one technique is particularly helpful for adults. Brainstorm a list of topics, and write each one on a separate index card. Then, every tutoring session, take turns selecting a topic on which you both will write. Write for ten minutes or so and then share your writing. This technique is most helpful if your topics are far-fetched, even silly; for example, "the life of the penguin," or "Brussels sprouts: the maligned vegetable." Practicing with topics of this type, which neither you nor your student probably knows much about, can help create a lighter touch for writing.

If your student does not know how to type, it's recommended that she learn to do so. The program *Keyboarding Skills: All Grades* by Diana Hanbury King (Educators Publishing Service, Inc., 1986) is recommended. This program teaches where the home keys are, and then has students learn the letters by following the alphabet. Therefore, they first learn "a" and "b," and then "c," "d," and "e." This program really works for the adult with dyslexia. It is much faster and more effective than the programs that teach the letters by following the home keys, "a," "s," "d," "f," and so forth.

Issues Involved in Teaching Math

Once again, check those early concepts. If your student does not know them, teach them using manipulatives and the same principles of instruction that you use with younger students. With adults, it's important to discuss how they feel about working on such "basic" things. If you discuss this honestly and provide a private place for instruction, most adults are relieved to finally be learning something that they have had to pretend to know all these years.

Be sensitive about the manipulatives you use. Sometimes, if the objects appear too childlike, you can spray paint them all one color. This often makes them seem more appropriate for adults.

COLLEGE

Many students with dyslexia are very successful at college. Some go on to graduate school. In college, the student with dyslexia is finally able to choose her own area of interest. She is able to have flexibility in scheduling and course selection. Often, in this setting, her strengths begin to show more clearly, and she demonstrates great originality of thinking and other important strengths.

Many colleges have programs designed for the student with dyslexia. These programs provide a range of services, from tutoring help for specific classes to a clinic setting where students can go for more remedial help. There are also colleges that are specifically designed for the student with dyslexia. A student can choose the type of setting she needs based on her academic needs and, also, on what she wants to study and where that is available.

The following suggestions can be given to the student with dyslexia for making college a successful and enjoyable experience:

Consider taking a lighter load than the "normal" 12 or 15 credits a semester. This is particularly helpful if reading speed or writing speed is somewhat slow. Also, because part of the dyslexic learning style is to be intensely curious about a topic that is interesting, it may suit the student more to be able to focus on fewer subjects and to delve deeply into them.

In any given semester, consider taking courses that are related to one another. As people with dyslexia tend to think globally and enjoy discovering patterns and underlying concepts, it can be interesting for them to focus in a particular intellectual area, for example, "Medieval Art" and "Literature in the Medieval Period." The commonality here is the medieval time. The student with dyslexia can appreciate learning about many aspects of life in one period.

Consider asking for accommodations such as the following:

- A tape recorder to tape lectures
- Peer support for sharing lecture notes
- Support with grammar and spelling when writing papers
- Support with organizing papers and projects
- Support with organizing time
- Support with computer skills
- Untimed or time-and-a-half testing
- Oral testing
- The waiving of, or substitution option for, a foreign language requirement

Consider using recorded textbooks. The recommended way to use these recordings is to play the tape while reading the print. In this way, visual and auditory skills interact to help increase speed of reading. This technique also assists reading comprehension. These taped books can be obtained from an organization called Recordings for the Blind and Dyslexic. More information on this group is provided in Chapter 17 of this resource.

If a foreign language requirement is not waived, choose the language to be studied very carefully. Usually, either Latin or Spanish is recommended. Latin is suggested because of its high degree of structure. It also gives the student useful information about the English language. Spanish is often recommended because it is phonetically regular.

In some colleges, sign language is now being offered as a language to study. This can be an excellent option for some students, especially those with good bodily-kinesthetic intelligence. It is often suggested that students not study French because of the many phonetic irregularities in the language.

As important as it is to select the language carefully, it is also helpful to ask about the teaching style that is used in individual classes. As with other subjects, students with dyslexia tend to learn languages most easily when classes are structured, when material is presented in small, sequential units, when there is much opportunity for review and practice, and when multimodalities are utilized.

Check out published resources. An excellent pamphlet is *College: How Students with Dyslexia Can Maximize the Experience* by Joan Stoner, Mary L. Farrell, and Barbara Priddy Guyer (The Orton Dyslexia Society, 1996). This monograph covers in more detail the basic points discussed above and also presents other issues relating to college. It is strongly recommended as a small book to start with for the student who is thinking of going to college.

IN CONCLUSION

Teaching adults with dyslexia can be a fascinating and extremely rewarding experience. Also, having insight into the learning style of adult family members of your younger students is very helpful. Your ability to relate to them in a positive and supportive way will help you be more effective in working with their children.

As we come to understand this fascinating learning style more and more, we are discovering that there are fewer artificial limits than there were in the past. Students with dyslexia of all ages, from infants to adults, can learn. When provided with appropriate intervention, they can succeed with academics. Then, they can utilize their talents, and they can offer much to the world.

BIBLIOGRAPHY

ADD/ADHD Behavior-Change Resource Kit: Ready-to-Use Strategies and Activities for Helping Children with Attention Deficit Disorder by Grad L. Flick, Ph.D. (The Center for Applied Research in Education, 1998)

The ADD/ADHD Checklist: An Easy Reference for Parents and Teachers by Sandra Rief, M.A. (Prentice Hall, 1998)

Attack Math: Arithmetic Tasks to Advance Computational Knowledge by Carole Greenes, George Immerzeel, Linda Schulman, Rika Spungin (Educators Publishing Service, Inc., 1985)

Basic Montessori, Learning Activities for Under-Fives by David Gettman (St. Martin's Press, 1987)

Beginning Connected: Cursive Handwriting, (The Johnson Handwriting Program), by Warren T. Johnson and Mary R. Johnson, Educators Publishing Service, Inc., 1961, 1963, 1971, 1972, 1976)

Beyond Ritalin: Facts About Medication and Other Strategies for Helping Children, Adolescents and Adults with Attention Deficit Disorders by Stephen W. Garber, PH.D., Marianne Daniels Garber, PH.D., and Robyn Freedman Spizman (Harper Perennial, copyright 1996 by Marianne Garber, Ph.D, Stephen W. Garber, Ph.D. and Robyn Freedman Spizman).

Cursive Writing Skills by Diana Hanbury King (Educators Publishing Service, Inc., 1987)

Developing Independent Readers: Strategy-Oriented Reading Activities for Learners with Special Needs by Cynthia Conway Waring (The Center for Applied Research in Education, 1995)

Developing Letter-Sound Connections: A Strategy-Oriented Alphabet Activities Program for Beginning Readers and Writers by Cynthia Conway Waring (Center for Applied Research in Education, 1998)

Dyslexia: Research and Resource Guide by Carol Sullivan Spafford and George S. Grosser (Allyn and Bacon, 1996)

Dyslexia: Theory and Practice of Remedial Instruction, Second Edition, by Diana Brewster Clark and Joanna Kellogg Uhry (York Press, 1995)

Family Math by Jean Kerr Stenmark, Virginia Thompson and Ruth Cossey, illustrated by Marilyn Hill (The Lawrence Hall of Science, 1986 by the Regents, University of California)

Finding Help When Your Child is Struggling in School, From Kindergarten Through Junior High School, by Lawrence J. Greene (Golden Books, 1998)

Frames of Mind: The Theory of Multiple Intelligences by Howard Gardner (Basic Books, 1983)

How to Reach and Teach ADD/ADHD Children: Practical Techniques, Strategies, and Interventions for Helping Children with Attention Problems and Hyperactivity by Sandra F. Rief (The Center for Applied Research in Education, 1993)

In The Mind's Eye: Visual Thinkers, Gifted People With Dyslexia And Other Learning Difficulties, Computer Images And The Ironies of Creativity by Thomas G. West (Prometheus Books, 1997)

Keyboarding Skills by Diana Hanbury King (Educators Publishing Service, Inc., 1988)

The Kim Marshall Series in Reading by Kim Marshall (Educators Publishing Service, Inc., 1984, 1982)

The Kim Marshall Series: Math, Parts A and B by Kim Marshall (Educators Publishing Service, Inc., *Part A*: 1982, 1984, 1997, *Part B*: 1983)

The LD Child and the ADHD Child: Ways Parents and Professionals Can Help by Suzanne H. Stevens (John F. Blair, Publisher, Winston-Salem, NC, 1996)

Learning Disabilities and the Law by Peter S. Latham, J.D. and Patricia H. Latham, J.D. (JKL Communications, Washington, D.C., 1993)

Let's Write! A Ready-to-Use Activities Program for Learners with Special Needs by Cynthia M. Stowe (The Center For Applied Research in Education, 1997)

Lindamood Phoneme Sequencing Program (formerly known as the *A.D.D. Program, Auditory Discrimination in Depth*) by Charles H. Lindamood and Patricia C. Lindamood (DLM Teaching Resources, 1969, 1975)

Mathematics Their Way by Mary Baretta-Lorton (Addison-Wesley, 1976)

Mathematics: A Way of Thinking by Robert Baretta-Lorton (Addison Wesley Publishing, 1977)

A Montessori Handbook: "Dr. Montessori's Own Handbook" With Additional New Material on Current Montessori Theory and Practice, Edited by R.C. Orem (G.P. Putnam's Sons, 1965)

Multisensory Teaching Approach (MTA) Handwriting Program by Margaret Taylor Smith (Educators Publishing Service, Inc., 1987, 1988)

Negotiating the Special Education Maze: A Guide for Parents and Teachers, Third Edition by Winifred Anderson, Stephen Chitwood and Deidre Hayden (Woodbine House, 1997)

On Cloud Nine, Visualizing and Verbalizing for Math by Kimberly Tuley and Nanci Bell (Gander Publishing, 1997)

The PAF Handwriting Program by Phyllis Bertin and Eileen Perlman (Educators Publishing Service, Inc., 1997, 1995)

Power Parenting for Children with ADD/ADHD: A Practical Parent's Guide for Managing Difficult Behaviors by Grad L. Flick, Ph.D., (The Center for Applied Research in Education, West Nyack, New York, 1996)

Reading Stories for Comprehension Success: 45 High-Interest Lessons with Reproducible Selections and Questions That Make Kids Think, Vol. 1: Primary Level, Grades 1-3, Vol. 2: Intermediate Level, Grades 4-6, Junior High Level, Grades 7-9 by Katherine L. Hall (The Center for Applied Research in Education, 1996, 1999)

Reading for Understanding by Thelma Gwinn Thurstone (Science Research Associates, Inc., 1978)

Reading Comprehension in Varied Subject Matter by Jane Ervin (Educators Publishing Service, Inc., 1970–1993)

Reversals: A Personal Account of Victory Over Dyslexia by Eileen Simpson (Houghton Mifflin Company, 1979).

Seeing Stars: Symbol Imagery for Phonemic Awareness, Sight Words and Spelling by Nanci Bell (Gander Publishing, 1997)

Spelling Smart! A Ready-to-Use Activities Program for Students with Spelling Difficulties by Cynthia M. Stowe (The Center for Applied Research in Education, 1996)

Structures and Techniques: Multisensory Teaching Of Basic Language Skills by Aylet R. Cox (Educators Publishing Service, Inc., 1984, 1980, 1977, 1975, 1974, 1969, 1967)

Visualizing and Verbalizing for Language Comprehension and Thinking by Nanci Bell (Academy of Reading Publications, 1986, 1991)

OTHER:

(article) *"Literacy Development in Successful Men and Women with Dyslexia"* by Rosalie P. Fink, Lesley College, in the *Annals of Dyslexia, An Interdisciplinary Journal of The International Dyslexia Association, Founded in memory of Samuel T. Orton, Volume XLVIII,* pp. 311-346 (The International Dyslexia Association, 1998)

(booklet) *College: How Students with Dyslexia Can Maximize the Experience* by Joan Stoner, Mary L. Farrell and Barbara Priddy Guyer (The Orton Dyslexia Society, 1996)